comprehensive
PART I
examination

The National Medical Series for Independent Study

review for national board comprehensive
PART I
examination

John S. Lazo, Ph.D.

Chairman, Department of Pharmacology
Allegheny Foundation Professor of Pharmacology
University of Pittsburgh
  School of Medicine
Pittsburgh, Pennsylvania

Bruce R. Pitt, Ph.D.

Vice Chairman, Department of Pharmacology
Professor of Pharmacology
  and Anesthesiology
University of Pittsburgh
  School of Medicine
Pittsburgh, Pennsylvania

Joseph C. Glorioso, III, Ph.D.

Chairman, Department of Molecular
  Genetics and Biochemistry
William S. McEllroy Professor of
  Biochemistry
University of Pittsburgh
  School of Medicine
Pittsburgh, Pennsylvania

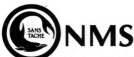

National Medical Series from Williams & Wilkins
Baltimore, Hong Kong, London, Sydney

Harwal Publishing Company, Media, Pennsylvania

Williams & Wilkins

Editorial management, production, and art direction: Jane Velker, Donna Rae Male
Acquisitions editor: J. Matthew Harris

The authors and publisher acknowledge with appreciation the use of questions from NMS books that exemplify the integrated format of the new examination.

The following illustrations have been reprinted with permission from the National Medical Series for Independent Study, Baltimore, Williams & Wilkins:
Figure 171–175 from April EW: *Anatomy*, 2nd edition, 1990
Figures 61, 110, 146, 151 from Bullock J, Boyle J, Wang MB, et al: *Physiology,* 1984
Figures 1, 92, 112, 159 from Bullock J, Boyle J, Wang MB: *Physiology,* 2nd edition, 1991
Figures 32–34, 192–194, 215–218, 237–241 from Johnson KE: *Histology and Cell Biology,* 2nd edition, 1991
Figure 211–215 from Johnson KE: *Human Developmental Anatomy,* 1988

Figure 43–44 has been reprinted with permission from Bates DV, Macklem PT, Christie RV: *Respiratory Function in Disease*, 2nd edition, Philadelphia, WB Saunders, 1971.
Figure 68–70 has been reprinted with permission from West JB: *Pulmonary Pathophysiology*, 3rd edition, Baltimore, Williams & Wilkins, 1987.
Figure 91 has been reprinted with permission from Gilman AG, Rau TW, Nies AS, et al: Goodman and Gilman's *The Pharmacological Basis of Therapeutics*, 8th edition, Elmsford, New York, Pergamon Press, 1990.
Figure 97 has been reprinted with permission from Murray J: *The Normal Lung*, Philadelphia, WB Saunders, 1976.

Library of Congress Cataloging-in Publication Data

Lazo, John S.
    Review for national board comprehensive part I examination / John S. Lazo, Bruce R. Pitt, Joseph C. Glorioso, III.
      p.   cm. — (The National medical series for independent study) ISBN 0-683-06213-1 (pbk. alk. paper)
    1. Medicine—Examinations, questions, etc. I. Glorioso, Joseph C. II. Pitt, Bruce R. III. Title. IV Series.
    [DNLM: 1. Medicine—examination questions. 2. Medicine—outlines. W 18 L431r]
R834.5.L39 1991
610'.76—dc20
DNLM/DLC
for Library of Congress   91-11949
                                                              CIP
ISBN 0-683-06213-1

© 1991 by Williams & Wilkins, Baltimore, Maryland

Printed in the United States of America. All rights reserved. Except as permitted under the Copyright Act of 1976, no part of this Publication may be reproduced or distributed in any form or by any means or stored in a data base or retrieval system, without the prior written permission of the publisher.

10 9 8 7 6 5 4 3 2 1

Dedication

To Jacqui, Shayna, and Stacy

Contents

Preface — ix

Acknowledgments — xi

Publisher's Note — xiii

Taking a Test — xv

Practice Examination I
  Questions — 1
  Answer Key — 33
  Answers and Explanations — 35

Practice Examination II
  Questions — 61
  Answer Key — 99
  Answers and Explanations — 101

Contents

Preface	ix
Acknowledgments	xi
Publisher's Note	xiii
Taking a Test	xv
Practice Examination I	
Questions	1
Answer Key	33
Answers and Explanations	35
Practice Examination II	
Questions	61
Answer Key	99
Answers and Explanations	101

Preface

Much like the events that took place during the first quarter of this century, there are major changes currently occurring in the approach to medical education in the United States. There have been rapid advances in our understanding of the molecular basis of diseases; an enormous increase in the data that can be presented to medical students; and a consolidation of experimental methodologies in the basic sciences. As a result, there is now a general consensus that a greater emphasis should be placed on an integrated presentation of information during the first 2 years of medical school.

Few institutions provide students with a comprehensive examination that will test their grasp of the key concepts presented in their first 2 years of medical school. With the advent of a new Part I National Board examination that de-emphasizes the traditional basic science disciplines and stresses the integrated approach, we believe it is especially important to provide students with a series of questions that will prepare them for this new format. We hope you will find this book useful, and we, as well as the publisher, welcome any comments you may have.

John S. Lazo
Bruce R. Pitt
Joseph C. Glorioso, III

Acknowledgments

The writing of this book could not have been accomplished without the tremendous assistance of many individuals in the Departments of Pharmacology, Molecular Genetics and Biochemistry, and Human Genetics at the University of Pittsburgh. Particular thanks are extended to Drs. R. R. Bahnson, J. Barranger, C. Coffee, D. Edelstone, D. Feingold, W. F. Goins, E. P. Hoffman, S. Kaplan, M. Lotze, B. McClane, T. Mietzner, C. Milcarek, G. Morris, K. Norris, B. Phillips, S. Phillips, F. Ruben, and D. Tweardy. We also wish to acknowledge the contributions of John Mignano, Theresa Hartsell, and James Rusnack, who are second-year medical students at the University of Pittsburgh, and Sharon Webb, for her secretarial support. Finally, this book could not have been successfully published without the thoughtful and tireless assistance of Jane Velker and Donna Male at Harwal Publishing.

Publisher's Note

In 1983, the National Board of Medical Examiners created a study committee to review the format of the National Board exam and to evaluate its effectiveness vis-à-vis the current state of medical education. The committee identified a number of deficiencies in format and made some sweeping recommendations on how to improve the exam. In 1986, following the recommendations of the committee, the National Board appointed Comprehensive Part I and Comprehensive Part II committees and charged them with the responsibility of creating new examinations. The results are the National Board Comprehensive Part I and Part II exams. The Part I exam will be introduced in June 1991.

The comprehensive exam differs from the old exam in both intent and format. The intent is best described by *The Medical Board Examiner* (Winter 1990).

(The new exam is) designed to be a broadly based, integrated examination for certification, rather than distinct achievement tests in individual basic science disciplines. Emphasis is on basic biomedical science concepts deemed important as part of the foundation for the current and future practice of medicine, including those related to the prevention of disease.

The format has been modified to reflect the objectives of the comprehensive exam. Concepts and information tested will remain the same but will be presented in a different framework. The new exam will continue to use questions drawn from single disciplines but will also include questions designed to test whether the examinee understands and can apply concepts of basic biomedical science in an integrated, cross-discipline manner. Case studies, or vignettes, will serve as clinical foundations for this approach.

The books in the National Medical Series have always been exceptional sources of information for medical students. By using the narrative outline, the books facilitate learning a large amount of information in a short period of time. Whether they are used for course study, exam preparation, or Board review, the NMS books will continue to offer medical students a reliable low-cost way to excel.

This new book on the NMS list is intended to be used along with the other NMS books and to help medical students:

- prepare for the new Comprehensive Part I exam by reviewing all of the major content areas covered on the exam
- become acquainted and comfortable with the new exam format
- determine areas where they may need further study through the use of the key concepts included at the beginning of each explanation

Use this book along with other material as you prepare for the exam. The authors and publisher have made every effort to ensure that all of the information in this book is accurate. Best of luck.

The Publisher

Taking a Test

One of the least attractive aspects of pursuing an education is the necessity of being examined on what has been learned. Instructors do not like to prepare tests, and students do not like to take them.

However, students are required to take many examinations during their learning careers, and little if any time is spent acquainting them with the positive aspects of tests and with systematic and successful methods for approaching them. Students perceive tests as punitive and sometimes feel that they are merely opportunities for the instructor to discover what the student has forgotten or has never learned. Students need to view tests as opportunities to display their knowledge and to use them as tools for developing prescriptions for further study and learning.

A brief history and discussion of the National Board of Medical Examiners (NBME) examinations (i.e., Parts I, II, and III and FLEX) are presented here, along with ideas concerning psychological preparation for the examinations. Also presented are general considerations and test-taking tips, as well as ways to use practice exams as educational tools. (The literature provided by the various examination boards contains detailed information concerning the construction and scoring of specific exams.)

National Board of Medical Examiners Examinations

Before the various NBME exams were developed, each state attempted to license physicians through its own procedures. Differences between the quality and testing procedures of the various state examinations resulted in the refusal of some states to recognize the licensure of physicians licensed in other states. This made it difficult for physicians to move freely from one state to another and produced an uneven quality of medical care in the United States.

To remedy this situation, the various state medical boards decided they would be better served if an outside agency prepared standard exams to be given in all states, allowing each state to meet its own needs and have a common standard by which to judge the educational preparation of individuals applying for licensure.

One misconception concerning these outside agencies is that they are licensing authorities. This is not the case; they are examination boards only. The individual states retain the power to grant and revoke licenses. The examination boards are charged with designing and scoring valid and reliable tests. They are primarily concerned with providing the states with feedback on how examinees have performed and with making suggestions about the interpretation and usefulness of scores. The states use this information as partial fulfillment of qualifications upon which they grant licenses.

The author of this introduction, Michael J. O'Donnell, holds the positions of Assistant Professor of Psychiatry and Director of Biomedical Communications at the University of New Mexico School of Medicine, Albuquerque, New Mexico.

Students should remember that these exams are administered nationwide and, although the general medical information is the same, educational methodologies and faculty areas of expertise differ from institution to institution. It is unrealistic to expect that students will know all the material presented in the exams; they may face questions on the exams in areas that were only superficially covered in their classes. The testing authorities recognize this situation, and their scoring procedures take it into account.

The Exams

The first exam was given in 1916. It was a combination of written, oral, and laboratory tests, and it was administered over a 5-day period. Admission to the exam required proof of completion of medical education and 1 year of internship.

In 1922, the examination was changed to a new format and was divided into three parts. Part I, a 3-day essay exam, was given in the basic sciences after 2 years of medical school. Part II, a 2-day exam, was administered shortly before or after graduation, and Part III was taken at the end of the first postgraduate year. To pass both Part I and Part II, a score equaling 75% of the total points available in each was required.

In 1954, after a 3-year extensive study, the NBME adopted the multiple-choice format. To pass, a statistically computed score of 75 was required, which allowed comparison of test results from year to year. In 1971, this method was changed to one that held the mean constant at a computed score of 500, with a predetermined deviation from the mean to ascertain a passing or failing score. The 1971 changes permitted more sophisticated analysis of test results and allowed schools to compare among individual students within their respective institutions as well as among students nationwide. Feedback to students regarding performance included the reporting of pass or failure along with scores in each of the areas tested.

During the 1980s, the ever-changing field of medicine made it necessary for the NBME to examine once again its evaluation strategies. It was found necessary to develop questions in multidisciplinary areas such as gerontology, health promotion, immunology, and cell and molecular biology. In addition, it was decided that questions should test higher cognitive levels and reasoning skills.

To meet the new goals, many changes have been made in both the form and content of the examination. These changes include reduction in the number of questions to approximately 800 in Part I and Part II to allow students more time on each question, with total testing time reduced on Part I from 13 to 12 hours and on Part II from 12.5 to 12 hours. The basic science disciplines are no longer allotted the same number of questions, which permits flexible weighing of the exam areas. Reporting of scores to schools includes total scores for individuals and group mean scores for separate discipline areas. Only pass/fail designations and total scores are reported to examinees. There is no longer a provision for the reporting of individual subscores to either the examinees or medical schools. Finally, the question format used in the new exams, now referred to as Comprehensive (Comp) I and II, is predominantly multiple-choice, best-answer.

The New Format

New questions, designed specifically for Comp I, are constructed in an effort to test the student's grasp of the sciences basic to medicine in an integrated fashion— the questions are designed to be interdisciplinary. Many of these items are presented as vignettes, or case studies, followed by a series of multiple-choice, best-answer questions.

The scoring of this exam is altered. Whereas in the past the exams were scored on a normal curve, the new exam has a predetermined standard, which must be met in order to pass. The exam no longer concentrates on the trivial; therefore, it has been concluded that there is a common base of information that all medical students should know in order to pass. It is anticipated that a major shift in the pass/fail rate for the nation is unlikely. In the past, the average student could only expect to feel comfortable with half the test and eventually would complete approximately 67% of the questions correctly, to achieve a mean score of 500. Although with the standard setting method it is likely that the mean score will change and become higher, it is unlikely that the pass/fail rates will differ significantly from those in the past. During the first testing in 1991, there will not be differential weighing of questions. However, in the future, the NBME will be researching methods of weighing questions based on both the time it takes to answer questions vis-à-vis their difficulty and the perceived importance of the information. In addition, the NBME is attempting to design a method of delivering feedback to the student that will have considerable importance in discovering weaknesses and pinpointing areas for further study in the event that a retake is necessary.

Since many of the proposed changes will be implemented for the first time in June 1991, specific information regarding actual standards, question emphasis, pass/fail rates, and so forth were unavailable at the time of publication. The publisher will update this section as information becomes available and as we attempt to follow the evolution and changes that occur in the area of physician evaluation.

Materials Needed for Test Preparation

In preparation for a test, many students collect far too much study material only to find that they simply do not have the time to go through all of it. They are defeated before they begin because either they leave areas unstudied, or they race through the material so quickly that they cannot benefit from the activity.

It is generally more efficient for the student to use materials already at hand; that is, class notes, one good outline to cover or strengthen areas not locally stressed and to quickly review the whole topic, and one good text as a reference for looking up complex material needing further explanation.

Also, many students attempt to memorize far too much information, rather than learning and understanding less material and then relying on that learned information to determine the answers to questions at the time of the examination. Relying too heavily on memorized material causes anxiety, and the more anxious students become during a test, the less learned knowledge they are likely to use.

Positive Attitude

A positive attitude and a realistic approach are essential to successful test taking. If concentration is placed on the negative aspects of tests or on the potential for failure, anxiety increases and performance decreases. A negative attitude generally develops if the student concentrates on "I must pass" rather than on "I can pass." "What if I fail?" becomes the major factor motivating the student to **run from failure rather than toward success.** This results from placing too much emphasis on scores rather than understanding that scores have only slight relevance to future professional performance.

The score received is only one aspect of test performance. Test performance also indicates the student's ability to use information during evaluation procedures and reveals how this ability might be used in the future. For example, when a patient enters the physician's office with a problem, the physician begins by asking questions, searching for clues, and seeking diagnostic information. Hypotheses are then developed, which will include several potential causes for the problem. Weighing the probabilities, the physician will begin to discard those hypotheses with the least likelihood of being correct. Good differential diagnosis involves the ability to deal with uncertainty, to reduce potential causes to the smallest number, and to use all learned information in arriving at a conclusion.

The same thought process can and should be used in testing situations. It might be termed **paper-and-pencil differential diagnosis.** In each question with five alternatives, of which one is correct, there are four alternatives that are incorrect. If deductive reasoning is used, as in solving a clinical problem, the choices can be viewed as having possibilities of being correct. The elimination of wrong choices increases the odds that a student will be able to recognize the correct choice. Even if the correct choice does not become evident, the probability of guessing correctly increases. Just as differential diagnosis in a clinical setting can result in a correct diagnosis, eliminating choices on a test can result in choosing the correct answer.

Answering questions based on what is incorrect is difficult for many students since they have had nearly 20 years experience taking tests with the implied assertion that knowledge can be displayed only by knowing what is correct. It must be remembered, however, that students can display knowledge by knowing something is wrong, just as they can display it by knowing something is right. **Students should begin to think in the present as they expect themselves to think in the future.**

Paper-and-Pencil Differential Diagnosis

The technique used to arrive at the answer to the following question is an example of the paper-and-pencil differential diagnosis approach.

A recently diagnosed case of hypothyroidism in a 45-year-old man may result in which of the following conditions?

(A) Thyrotoxicosis
(B) Cretinism
(C) Myxedema
(D) Graves' disease
(E) Hashimoto's thyroiditis

It is presumed that all of the choices presented in the question are plausible and partially correct. If the student begins by breaking the question into parts and trying to discover what the question is attempting to measure, it will be possible to answer the question correctly by using more than memorized charts concerning thyroid problems.

- The question may be testing if the student knows the difference between "hypo" and "hyper" conditions.
- The answer choices may include thyroid problems that are not "hypothyroid" problems.
- It is possible that one or more of the choices are "hypo" but are not "thyroid" problems, that they are some other endocrine problems.
- "Recently diagnosed in a 45-year-old man" indicates that the correct answer is not a congenital childhood problem.
- "May result in" as opposed to "resulting from" suggests that the choices might include a problem that **causes** hypothyroidism rather than **results from** hypothyroidism, as stated.

By applying this kind of reasoning, the student can see that choice **A**, thyroid toxicosis, which is a disorder resulting from an overactive thyroid gland ("hyper") must be eliminated. Another piece of knowledge, that is, Graves' disease is thyroid toxicosis, eliminates choice **D**. Choice **B**, cretinism, is indeed hypothyroidism, but is a childhood disorder. Therefore, **B** is eliminated. Choice **E** is an inflammation of the thyroid gland—here the clue is the suffix "itis." The reasoning is that thyroiditis, being an inflammation, may **cause** a thyroid problem, perhaps even a hypothyroid problem, but there is no reason for the reverse to be true. Myxedema, choice **C**, is the only choice left and the obvious correct answer.

Preparing for Board Examinations

1. Study for yourself. Although some of the material may seem irrelevant, the more you learn now, the less you will have to learn later. Also, do not let the fear of the test rob you of an important part of your education. If you study to learn, the task is less distasteful than studying solely to pass a test.

2. Review all areas. You should not be selective by studying perceived weak areas and ignoring perceived strong areas. This is probably the last time you will have the time and the motivation to review **all** of the basic sciences.

3. Attempt to understand, not just memorize, the material. Ask yourself: To whom does the material apply? Where does it apply? When does it apply? Understanding the connections among these points allows for longer retention and aids in those situations when guessing strategies may be needed.

4. Try to **anticipate questions that might appear on the test.** Ask yourself how you might construct a question on a specific topic.

5. Give yourself a couple days of rest before the test. Studying up to the last moment will increase your anxiety and cause potential confusion.

Taking Board Examinations

1. In the case of NBME exams, be sure to **pace yourself** to use the time optimally. Each booklet is designed to take 2 hours. You should use all of your allotted time; if you finish too early, you probably did so by moving too quickly through the test.

2. Read each question and all the alternatives carefully before you begin to make decisions. Remember the questions contain clues, as do the answer choices. As a physician, you would not make a clinical decision without a complete examination of all the data: the same holds true for answering test questions.

3. Read the directions for each question set carefully. You would be amazed at how many students make mistakes in tests simply because they have not paid close attention to the directions.

4. It is not advisable to leave blanks with the intention of coming back to answer the questions later. Because of the way Board examinations are constructed, you probably will not pick up any new information that will help you when you come back, and the chances of getting numerically off on your answer sheet are greater than your chances of benefiting by skipping around. If you feel that you must come back to a question, mark the best choice and place a note in the margin. Generally speaking, it is best not to change answers once you have made a decision. Your intuitive reaction and first response are correct more often than changes made out of frustration or anxiety. **Never turn in an answer sheet with blanks.** Scores are based on the number that you get correct; you are not penalized for incorrect choices.

5. Do not try to answer the questions on a stimulus-response basis. It generally will not work. Use all of your learned knowledge.

6. Do not let anxiety destroy your confidence. If you have prepared conscientiously, you know enough to pass. Use all that you have learned.

7. Do not try to determine how well you are doing as you proceed. You will not be able to make an objective assessment, and your anxiety will increase.

8. Do not expect a feeling of mastery or anything close to what you are accustomed to. Remember, this is a nationally administered exam, not a mastery test.

9. Do not become frustrated or angry about what appear to be bad or difficult questions. You simply do not know the answers; you cannot know everything.

Specific Test-Taking Strategies

Read the entire question carefully, regardless of format. Test questions have multiple parts. Concentrate on picking out the pertinent key words that might help you begin to problem-solve. Words such as "always," "never," "mostly," "primarily," and so forth play significant roles. In all types of questions, distractors with terms such as "always" or "never" most often are incorrect. Adjectives and adverbs can completely change the meaning of questions—pay close attention to them. Also, medical prefixes and suffixes (e.g., "hypo-," "hyper-," "-ectomy," "-itis") are sometimes at the root of the question. The knowledge and application of everyday English grammar often is the key to dissecting questions.

Multiple-Choice Questions

Read the question and the choices carefully to become familiar with the data as given. Remember, in multiple-choice questions there is one correct answer and there are four distractors, or incorrect answers. (Distractors are plausible and possibly correct or they would not be called distractors.) They are generally correct for part of the question but not for the entire question. Dissecting the question into parts aids in discerning these distractors.

If the correct answer is not immediately evident, begin eliminating the distractors. (Many students feel that they must always start at option A and make a decision before they move to B, thus forcing decisions they are not ready to make.) Your first decisions should be made on those choices you feel the most confident about.

Compare the choices to each part of the question. **To be wrong,** a choice needs to be **incorrect for only part** of the question. **To be correct,** it must be **totally** correct. If you believe a choice is partially incorrect, tentatively eliminate that choice. Make notes next to the choices regarding tentative decisions. One method is to place a minus sign next to the choices you are certain are incorrect and a plus sign next to those that potentially are correct. Finally, place a zero next to any choice you do not understand or need to come back to for further inspection. Do not feel that you must make final decisions until you have examined all choices carefully.

When you have eliminated as many choices as you can, decide which of those that are left has the highest probability of being correct. Remember to use paper-and-pencil differential diagnosis. Above all, be honest with yourself. If you do not know the answer, eliminate as many choices as possible and choose reasonably.

Vignette-Based Questions

Vignette-based questions are nothing more than normal multiple-choice questions that use the same case, or grouped information, for setting the problem. The NBME has been researching question types that would test the student's grasp of the integrated medical basic sciences in a more cognitively complex fashion than can be accomplished with traditional testing formats. These questions allow the testing of information that is more medically relevant than memorized terminology.

It is important to realize that several questions, although grouped together and referring to one situation or vignette, are independent questions; that is, they are able to stand alone. Your inability to answer one question in a group should have no bearing on your ability to answer other questions in that group.

These are multiple-choice questions, and just as with single best-answer questions, you should use the paper-and-pencil differential diagnosis, as was described earlier.

Single Best-Answer–Matching Sets

Single best-answer–matching sets consist of a list of words or statements followed by several numbered items or statements. Be sure to pay attention to whether the choices can be used more than once, only once, or not at all. Consider each choice individually and carefully. Begin with those with which you are the most familiar. It is important always to break the statements and words into parts, as with all other question formats. **If a choice is only partially correct, then it is incorrect.**

Guessing

Nothing takes the place of a firm knowledge base, but with little information to work with, even after playing paper-and-pencil differential diagnosis, you may find it necessary to guess at the correct answer. A few simple rules can help increase your guessing accuracy. Always guess consistently if you have no idea what is correct; that is, after eliminating all that you can, make the choice that agrees with your intuition or choose the option closest to the top of the list that has not been eliminated as a potential answer.

When guessing at questions that present with choices in numerical form, you will often find the choices listed in ascending or descending order. It is generally not wise to guess the first or last alternative, since these are usually extreme values and are most likely incorrect.

Using the Comprehensive Exam to Learn

All too often, students do not take full advantage of practice exams. There is a tendency to complete the exam, score it, look up the correct answers to those questions missed, and then forget the entire thing.

In fact, great educational benefits can be derived if students would spend more time using practice tests as learning tools. As mentioned earlier, incorrect choices in test questions are plausible and partially correct or they would not fulfill their purpose as distractors. This means that it is just as beneficial to look up the incorrect choices as the correct choices to discover specifically why they are incorrect. In this way, it is possible to learn better test-taking skills as the subtlety of question construction is uncovered.

Additionally, it is advisable to go back and attempt to restructure each question to see if all the choices can be made correct by modifying the question. By doing this, four times as much will be learned. By all means, look up the right answer and explanation. Then, focus on each of the other choices and ask yourself under what conditions they might be correct. For example, the entire thrust of the sample question concerning hypothyroidism could be altered by changing the first few words to read:

"Hyperthyroidism recently discovered in..."
"Hypothyroidism prenatally occurring in..."
"Hypothyroidism resulting from..."

This question can be used to learn and understand thyroid problems in general, not only to memorize answers to specific questions.

In the practice exams that follow, every effort has been made to simulate the types of questions and the degree of question difficulty in the NBME Part I Comprehensive exam. While taking these exams, the student should attempt to create the testing conditions that might be experienced during actual testing situations. Approximately 1 minute should be allowed for each question, and the entire test should be finished before it is scored.

Summary

Ideally, examinations are designed to determine how much information students have learned and how that information is used in the successful completion of the examination. Students will be successful if these suggestions are followed:

- Develop a positive attitude and maintain that attitude.
- Be realistic in determining the amount of material you attempt to master and in the score you hope to attain.
- Read the directions for each type of question and the questions themselves closely and follow the directions carefully.
- Guess intelligently and consistently when guessing strategies must be used.
- Bring the paper-and-pencil differential diagnosis approach to each question in the examination.
- Use the test as an opportunity to display your knowledge and as a tool for developing prescriptions for further study and learning.

National Board examinations are not easy. They may be almost impossible for those who have unrealistic expectations or for those who allow misinformation concerning the exams to produce anxiety out of proportion to the task at hand. They are manageable if they are approached with a positive attitude and with consistent use of all the information that has been learned.

Michael J. O'Donnell

Practice Examination I

QUESTIONS

Directions: Each of the numbered items or incomplete statements in this section is followed by answers or by completions of the statement. Select the **one** lettered answer or completion that is **best** in each case.

1. An action potential recorded from a microelectrode inserted in a nerve fiber is illustrated in the figure below. Which of the following statements best describes the changes that take place during the action potential recorded by these electrodes?

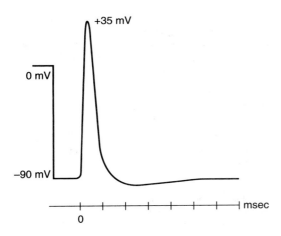

(A) At the peak of the action potential, the number of open Na⁺ channels equals the number of open K⁺ channels
(B) Depolarization is due to an abrupt increase in Na⁺ conductance
(C) Repolarization is primarily due to a decrease in K⁺ conductance
(D) Repolarization is due to activation of the Ca²⁺–Na⁺ channel
(E) Alteration in the permeability of chloride leak channels is generated by the action potential

2. A 24-year-old man presented to his family practitioner with a purulent penile discharge. Gonorrhea was diagnosed based upon the finding of intracellular gram-negative cocci in his discharge. He was given amoxicillin and probenecid. The infection improved, but 1 week later the patient still complained of a persistent urethral discharge and pain on urination. Upon a visit to a local clinic for sexually transmitted diseases, a diagnosis of postgonococcal urethritis was made. What is the most likely cause of his latest syndrome?

(A) A common side effect of probenecid administered during the initial treatment
(B) A lingering gonococcal infection caused by a penicillin-resistant strain of *Neisseria gonorrhoeae*
(C) An improper therapy regimen, which did not treat a coinciding chlamydial infection
(D) A side effect of the correct therapy regimen, which suppressed the patient's normal flora and allowed the establishment of a secondary infection

3. For which one of the following organisms do opsonic antibodies play a major role in acquired immunity to infection?

(A) *Neisseria meningitidis*, group A
(B) *Vibrio cholerae*
(C) *Clostridium botulinum*
(D) *Corynebacterium diphtheriae*

4. Each statement below concerning cyclic adenosine monophosphate (cAMP) is true EXCEPT

(A) cAMP levels may be increased or decreased by hormone stimulation
(B) it is the second messenger for the action of parathyroid hormone (PTH) on the kidney
(C) it activates protein kinase C by binding to the regulatory subunit and causing dissociation of the catalytic subunit
(D) it is degraded intracellularly by a family of phosphodiesterase isoenzymes
(E) it is synthesized from adenosine triphosphate (ATP)

Questions 5 and 6

Five percent of those comprising a particular population are known to carry a recessive gene for poliodystrophy, an inherited disorder characterized by the onset of recurrent seizures and dementia in early childhood. A 32-year-old woman who had a brother with this disorder seeks genetic counseling. The patient's husband, an only child, does not know if his family has a history of the disorder.

5. What is the probability that the patient is a carrier of poliodystrophy?

(A) 2/3
(B) 1/2
(C) 3/4
(D) 1/20
(E) 3/8

6. What is the probability that both the patient and her husband are carriers?

(A) 2/3
(B) 1/20
(C) 1/30
(D) 3/4
(E) 3/8

7. When comparing pertussis and diphtheria, true statements include which one of the following?

(A) Both pertussis and diphtheria are caused by bacteria that must adhere to respiratory tract cells
(B) Diphtheria symptoms are caused by an exotoxin, but no symptoms of pertussis result from an exotoxin
(C) The bacteria responsible for diphtheria and pertussis both produce endotoxin
(D) Pertussis is caused by an intracellular pathogen, but diphtheria is caused by an extracellular pathogen
(E) The neurologic problems observed with the current DPT vaccine are caused by the diphtheria component of this vaccine

8. The process of DNA replication can be best described by which of the following statements? DNA replication

(A) initiates at specific sites
(B) of the *Escherichia coli* chromosome starts at multiple origins
(C) is unidirectional for all DNAs
(D) is not dependent on the synthesis of RNA primers
(E) results in both strands of a daughter molecule being newly synthesized

9. A 100-year-old patient is observed to be tachypneic at 28 breaths per minute. Nurses record a normal body temperature. The clinician finds localized crackles in the right upper lobe. A chest radiograph is normal. What is the most logical explanation for these findings?

(A) Renal failure with volume overload
(B) Age-related changes in the respiratory tract
(C) Age-related neurologic change in the respiratory center set point
(D) Atelectatic crackles with resolution
(E) Pneumonia

10. Halothane has blood:gas and oil:gas partition coefficients of 2.4 and 220, respectively. Methoxyflurane has blood:gas and oil:gas coefficients of 13 and 950, respectively. Which of the following statements regarding these volatile anesthetics is correct?

(A) Both result in faster induction than nitrous oxide (blood:gas partition coefficient of 0.47)
(B) The minimal alveolar concentration of halothane is less than that of methoxyflurane
(C) Both agents are useful since they do not have any cardiodepressant effects
(D) Recovery from methoxyflurane is faster than that from halothane
(E) An increase in ventilatory rate makes the onset of anesthesia more rapid for either agent

11. According to the Henderson-Hasselbalch equation:

$$pH = 6.1 + \log [HCO_3^-]/0.03 \times P_{CO_2}$$

The apparent dissociation constant, pK', in blood is 6.1; and the solubility constant for CO_2 in plasma at 38° C is 0.03 mmol/L/mm Hg. If a patient has a plasma $[HCO_3^-]$ of 37 mmol/L and arterial P_{CO_2} of 60 mm Hg, then the patient is most likely to have (recall log 10 = 1; log 20 = 1.3; log 30 = 1.5; normal values of $[HCO_3^-]$ = 25 mmol/L; P_{CO_2} = 40 mm Hg)

(A) respiratory alkalosis
(B) respiratory acidosis
(C) fully compensated respiratory acidosis
(D) metabolic alkalosis
(E) metabolic acidosis

12. Which of the following structures contains Hassall's corpuscles?

(A) Thyroid gland
(B) Parathyroid gland
(C) Pineal gland
(D) Thymus
(E) Spleen

13. Baroreceptors are highly branched nerve endings, which generate receptor potentials that are proportional to the rate of change in arterial blood pressure; they can also adapt to changes in arterial blood pressure over a prolonged period of time (hours to days). Which of the following statements concerning the specific properties of baroreceptors is most accurate?

(A) Baroreceptors are important for long-term regulation of blood pressure
(B) Clamping both carotid arteries after cutting both vagus nerves results in a decrease in arterial blood pressure
(C) Massaging the carotid sinus area leads to bradycardia and a decrease in arterial blood pressure
(D) A decrease in blood pressure activates baroreceptors, which, in turn, directly activates the vasomotor center

14. Each of the following enzymes is essential for protecting red blood cells from the H_2O_2 (hydrogen peroxide) generated in vivo EXCEPT

(A) glutathione peroxidase
(B) 6-phosphogluconate dehydrogenase
(C) catalase
(D) transketolase
(E) glutathione reductase

15. All of the following nephritides are associated with hypocomplementemia EXCEPT

(A) immunoglobulin A nephropathy
(B) mesangioproliferative glomerulonephropathy
(C) serum sickness
(D) systemic lupus erythematosus
(E) vasculitis

16. Renal osteodystrophy is a condition that may follow chronic renal failure. Features of this condition include osteitis fibrosa cystica admixed with osteomalacia. The pathogenesis of this condition is characterized by all of the following EXCEPT

(A) phosphate retention and hyperphosphatemia
(B) low levels of 1,25-$(OH)_2D_3$ (calcitriol)
(C) elevated levels of calcitonin
(D) hyperparathyroidism
(E) hypocalcemia

17. A quantitative Gram stain revealed many fewer cells than expected from the turbidity of a bacterial culture. The decrease in cells was most likely due to

(A) inactivation of the cytochromes
(B) digestion of the bacterial cell wall by autolytic processes
(C) presence of gram-negative organisms in the culture
(D) presence of bacterial spores in the culture

18. The following sequence is a part of a globular protein. Which of the following statements best describes this peptide?

Ser-Val-Asp-Asp-Val-Phe-Ser-Glu-Val-Cys-His-Met-Arg

(A) At pH 7.4, the peptide has a net negative charge
(B) It has only one sulfur-containing amino acid
(C) The hydrophobic amino acid content exceeds the hydrophilic content
(D) Treatment with chymotrypsin would generate four smaller fragments
(E) Only three of the side chains are capable of forming hydrogen bonds

19. Which one of the following statements about energy storage and transfer is true?

(A) Adenosine triphosphate (ATP) can be synthesized from adenosine diphosphate (ADP) by phosphate transfer from 3-phosphoglycerate
(B) Phosphocreatine is an important energy source for muscle tissues
(C) Reactions that have a $K_{eq} > 1$ have a positive $\Delta G°$
(D) When ATP is hydrolyzed to adenosine monophosphate (AMP) and PP_i, the reaction is endergonic and will proceed spontaneously
(E) The energy of hydrolysis for phosphoenolpyruvate is less than that for pyrophosphate

20. The ability of erythrocytes to pump Na^+ from the cytoplasm into the plasma compartment would be compromised most directly by a total deficiency of

(A) 6-phosphogluconate dehydrogenase
(B) 1,3-diphosphoglycerate kinase
(C) pyruvate carboxylase
(D) glucose 6-phosphatase
(E) malate dehydrogenase

21. A 45-year-old woman has eaten some home-canned vegetables. Two days later she has blurred vision and difficulty swallowing. This is followed by respiratory distress and flaccid paralysis. The symptoms of her illness result from an intoxication caused by a bacterial toxin whose action involves which one of the following effects?

(A) ADP-ribosylation of elongation factor 2
(B) Blockage of release of inhibitory neurotransmitters
(C) Blockage of release of acetylcholine (ACh)
(D) Stimulation of adenylate cyclase to elevate intracellular cAMP levels
(E) Hemolysis resulting from sequestration of cholesterol in membranes

22. Of the following statements, which best describes integral membrane proteins? They

(A) have at least one α-helical domain of approximately 20 amino acids, which spans the bilayer
(B) are stabilized within the bilayer by a combination of hydrogen bonds and electrostatic interactions
(C) may be solubilized by altering the pH or the ionic strength
(D) are frequently glycoproteins in which the carbohydrate is on the cytosolic side of the membrane
(E) may display transverse movement in the lipid bilayer

23. Proof of the presence of active disease caused by *Mycobacterium tuberculosis* is provided by which one of the following diagnostic measures?

(A) The tuberculin test
(B) Clinical findings (e.g., weight loss, night sweats, cough, low-grade fever)
(C) Finding acid-fast organisms in sputum
(D) Isolation of *M. tuberculosis*

24. Each statement below concerning osteoclasts is true EXCEPT that they

(A) are found in Howship's lacuna
(B) resorb bone
(C) are stimulated by calcitonin
(D) are multinucleated
(E) help remodel bone

25. All of the following match important vasodilators with corresponding tissues EXCEPT

(A) adenosine — heart
(B) carbon dioxide — brain
(C) low oxygen — lung
(D) increased body temperature — skin

26. A lymph node removed from a 32-year-old man shows diffuse large cell lymphoma. Which of the following clinical scenarios most likely characterizes this patient?

(A) Disseminated disease at presentation, prolonged survival eventually succumbing to lymphoma or its complications
(B) Rapid development of circulating immature blasts requiring aggressive cytotoxic therapy
(C) > 90% chance of being alive 10 years after diagnosis
(D) Rapid death if therapy is unsuccessful, good chance for long-term survival if therapy achieves complete response
(E) Spontaneous remission in 20% of patients

27. According to the figure below, which one of the following conditions would result in a shift of the oxygen saturation curve from a to b?

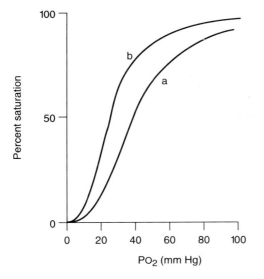

(A) A change in pH from 7.6 to 7.4
(B) A change in P_{CO_2} from 30 to 40 torrs
(C) An increase in the concentration of 2,3-diphosphoglycerate (DPG)
(D) The presence of fetal hemoglobin ($\alpha_2\gamma_2$)
(E) The oxidation of the heme iron from Fe^{2+} to Fe^{3+}

28. Tetracycline, a broad-spectrum antibiotic used in treating rickettsial, mycoplasmal, and chlamydial infections, receives widespread use because it

(A) is particularly useful in children
(B) causes minimal gastrointestinal side effects
(C) is bactericidal
(D) is selectively toxic to prokaryotes
(E) inhibits DNA-dependent RNA polymerase

29. Each statement below concerning fenestrated capillaries is true EXCEPT

(A) fenestrations are 60 nm to 100 nm in diameter
(B) they are present in the choroid plexus
(C) they may be partially surrounded by pericytes
(D) the slit diaphragm does not have a unit membrane structure
(E) the slit diaphragm forms a filtration barrier in the renal glomerulus

30. Propranolol (a β-blocker) may be used with nitroglycerin (glyceryl trinitrate; GTN) in concurrent therapy for typical (exertional) angina because propranolol

(A) is a potent vasodilator of coronary arteries
(B) increases conduction in the atria and atrioventricular node
(C) blocks the reflex tachycardia that occurs with the use of GTN
(D) dilates constricted airways
(E) is positively inotropic

31. A 20-year-old man has a penile lesion that is crateriform, moist, and indurated. The patient revealed that this lesion has been present for about 20 days and is not painful. Which one of the following groups of tests is most appropriate?

(A) Gram stain, Venereal Disease Research Laboratory (VDRL) test, and culture of lesion for *Treponema pallidum*
(B) Gram stain and culture of lesion for *T. pallidum*
(C) VDRL and darkfield examination
(D) Fluorescent treponemal antibody absorption (FTR-ABS) test

Questions 32–34

The micrograph below is taken from the male reproductive system.

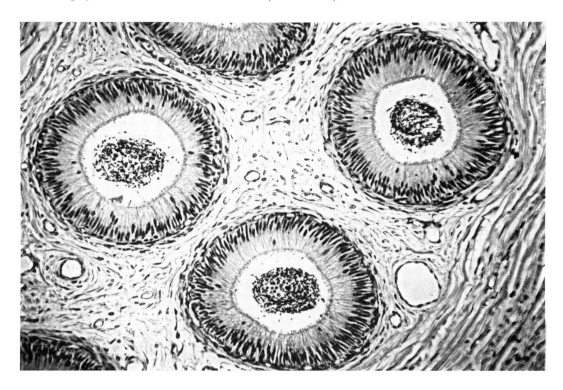

32. Which of the following organs is pictured in the micrograph?

(A) Testis
(B) Epididymis
(C) Vas deferens
(D) Seminal vesicle
(E) Bulbourethral gland

33. Which of the following epithelia best describes the epithelium of the organ in the micrograph?

(A) Simple cuboidal
(B) Simple columnar
(C) Stratified columnar
(D) Pseudostratified columnar with stereocilia
(E) Stratified squamous

34. Which phrase below best describes the function of the epithelium in the micrograph?

(A) Gametogenic
(B) Proliferative
(C) Secretory and absorptive
(D) Inactive
(E) Protective

35. The term that describes the adherence of neutrophils and monocytes to the vascular endothelium prior to movement into the extravascular space is

(A) margination
(B) diapedesis
(C) pavementing
(D) emigration
(E) clotting

36. Each condition below is a diagnostically significant abnormality in Zellweger syndrome EXCEPT

(A) absent or grossly reduced numbers of peroxisomes
(B) catalase in the cytosol of hepatocytes
(C) overproduction of platelet activating factor
(D) elevated plasma C26:0/C22:0 ratio
(E) accumulation of phytanic acid in central nervous system (CNS) tissues

37. A hospitalized patient is noted to have a urinary tract infection due to *Serratia*. A course of antimicrobial therapy with an aminoglycoside is planned. However, the patient is noted to have mild renal impairment. The best means to determine the appropriate drug dosage is

(A) body surface area
(B) serum creatinine
(C) serum blood urea nitrogen
(D) creatinine clearance
(E) peak and trough drug levels

38. An individual with a gastric carcinoma is likely to present with any of the following skin lesions EXCEPT

(A) seborrheic keratosis
(B) acanthosis nigricans
(C) erythema nodosum
(D) amyloidosis
(E) Paget's disease

39. The following elements of the adult brain develop from the telencephalon EXCEPT the

(A) corpus striatum
(B) internal capsule
(C) occipital lobe
(D) hippocampus
(E) thalamus

40. Which one of the following muscles raises the soft palate during swallowing?

(A) Levator veli palatini
(B) Palatoglossus
(C) Palatopharyngeus
(D) Superior constrictor

41. All of the following statements about hormone receptors are true EXCEPT that they

(A) may elicit their biologic response without being fully saturated with hormone
(B) may be desensitized by phosphorylation
(C) determine the specificity of cellular responses to hormones
(D) are deficient in Addison's disease
(E) are frequently transmembrane proteins

42. Asthma is characterized by an increased responsiveness of the trachea and bronchi to various stimuli and is manifested by widespread narrowing of the airway. Results of pulmonary function tests during an acute asthma attack will demonstrate all of the following EXCEPT

(A) decreased forced expiratory volume in 1 second (FEV_1)
(B) increased forced vital capacity (FVC)
(C) decreased FEV_1/FVC
(D) normal or increased total lung capacity (TLC)

43. All of the following statements about the peptide bond are true EXCEPT the

(A) peptide bond is planar
(B) peptide bond has restricted rotation
(C) α-carbon atoms are in a trans configuration
(D) peptide bond atoms do not participate in the secondary structure of proteins
(E) peptide bond has no charge associated with it

44. Of the following cell types, which would contain many mitochondria in the apical portion of the cell?

(A) Smooth muscle cells
(B) Ciliated cells
(C) Steroid-secreting cells
(D) Liver parenchymal cells
(E) Skeletal muscle cells

Questions 45 and 46

A 22-year-old male college student visits the student health service complaining of extreme fatigue, sore throat, difficulty concentrating, and fever to 39° C over the last week. Physical examination is unremarkable except for mild lymph node enlargement in axillary, cervical, and inguinal regions and a palpable spleen tip. A blood count shows hemoglobin of 10 g/dl, platelets of 105,000/μl, and white cell count of 22,000/μl with 60% lymphoid cells. The laboratory blood profile also shows an absolute red cell count of 2.3 x 10^6/μl, mean red cell volume (MCV) of 125 femtoliters (fl), and mean cell hemoglobin concentration of 43 g/dl.

45. What is the most likely diagnosis for this patient?

(A) Infectious lymphocytosis
(B) *Bordetella pertussis* infection
(C) Cytomegalovirus mononucleosis syndrome
(D) Mononucleosis secondary to Epstein-Barr virus (EBV) infection (infectious mononucleosis)
(E) Mononucleosis secondary to *Toxoplasma gondii* infection

46. For the patient described, which of the following is the most likely etiology for anemia (Hb 10 g/dl)?

(A) Immune-mediated
(B) Compromise of erythroid production secondary to EBV infection of bone marrow precursors
(C) Virus-associated hemophagocytic syndrome
(D) Slow gastrointestinal blood loss since the start of illness due to thrombocytopenia
(E) Disseminated intravascular coagulation (DIC)

47. All of the following statements concerning the major determinants of glomerular filtration rate (GFR), which are renal blood flow (RBF) and glomerular hydrostatic pressures, are correct EXCEPT

(A) constriction of the afferent arteriole decreases both RBF and GFR
(B) an increase in RBF, even with little change in glomerular pressure, increases GFR
(C) in a normal kidney, an increase in systemic arterial pressure from 100 to 150 mm Hg increases GFR severalfold
(D) constriction of the efferent arteriole decreases RBF and slightly increases GFR

48. A 65-year-old woman is seen prior to cataract surgery. She has had no previous surgery except for a dental extraction, after which she bled for 10 days and required a 2-unit blood transfusion. One sibling died from postoperative hemorrhage during childhood, and there is a history of bleeding in a number of relatives, both male and female. Her partial thromboplastin time (PTT) is markedly prolonged, and the bleeding time is within normal limits. The most likely diagnosis is

(A) factor VIII deficiency
(B) factor XI deficiency
(C) factor XII deficiency
(D) Fletcher factor deficiency
(E) von Willebrand's disease

49. A fecal specimen is cultured from a person with diarrhea, and *Shigella dysenteriae* and *Giardia lamblia* are isolated. All of the following statements about *Shigella* and *Giardia* are true EXCEPT

(A) *Shigella* has a peptidoglycan-containing cell wall but *G. lamblia* does not
(B) *Shigella* and *Giardia* both have DNA and RNA
(C) *Shigella* and *Giardia* both have sterol-containing plasma membranes
(D) *Shigella* has lipopolysaccharide but *Giardia* does not
(E) *Shigella* has 70S ribosomes but *Giardia* has 80S ribosomes

Questions 50–52

A resident has been assigned to the operating room for a 2-month rotation. The staff surgeon under whom he will work is a stickler for theory, and on the first day of the new rotation, he asked the resident the following questions.

50. With regard to anesthetics, MAC refers to

(A) maximum allowable concentration
(B) minimum alveolar concentration
(C) maximum alveolar concentration
(D) minimum arterial concentration
(E) maximum arterial concentration

51. If an anesthetic has a high blood:gas partition coefficient, it means that

(A) recovery will likely be prolonged
(B) lean patients should receive a lower dose than heavy patients
(C) the anesthetic should be delivered at a low concentration initially
(D) the anesthetic should be mixed with an inert gas or oxygen
(E) none of the above should occur

52. The molecular mechanism of action of anesthetic gases is

(A) increased solubility of membrane proteins
(B) increased mobility of membrane proteins
(C) increase in the molar volume of membrane phospholipids
(D) increase in membrane disorder (entropy)
(E) not known

53. Growth hormone (GH; somatotropic hormone; somatotropin) is synthesized and stored in large amounts in the anterior pituitary gland (adenohypophysis). Which of the following statements accurately describes growth hormone?

(A) It is secreted continuously
(B) Synthesis is stimulated by the action of somatostatin
(C) Receptors have a limited distribution outside the central nervous system
(D) It stimulates cartilage and bone growth via somatomedin
(E) It has a proinsulin-like effect in addition to its other actions

54. After osmotic equilibrium, infusion of several liters of a hypertonic saline solution will

(A) decrease intracellular osmolality
(B) not affect intracellular volume
(C) increase extracellular fluid volume
(D) decrease the plasma osmolarity

55. In a family with a disease that has an autosomal dominant inheritance pattern, seven children have been born, four of whom have the disease and three of whom do not. What is the probability of the next child born having the disease?

(A) 100%
(B) 50%
(C) 25%
(D) 0
(E) Cannot be determined

56. Which of the following tests is the major projective instrument of personality assessment?

(A) Rorschach Inkblot Test
(B) Minnesota Multiphasic Personality Inventory
(C) Thematic Apperception Test
(D) Sentence Completion Test
(E) Projective drawings

57. Synthesis of glycogen from fructose in a person with essential fructosuria requires the activity of which one of the following enzymes?

(A) Transketolase
(B) Aldolase B
(C) Hexokinase
(D) Fructokinase
(E) Glucokinase

58. Injection of a pharmacologically effective amount of an antimuscarinic agent, like atropine, may

(A) increase bronchial glandular secretions
(B) increase heart rate
(C) cause paralysis in some skeletal muscles
(D) constrict the pupil
(E) promote sweating

59. A very painful, spreading, cutaneous edematous erythema is clinically descriptive of

(A) erysipeloid
(B) diphtheria
(C) Pontiac fever
(D) listeriosis
(E) nocardiosis

60. A patient presents with a torn medial collateral ligament of the left knee. Which of the following signs may be elicited on physical examination?

(A) Posterior displacement of the tibia on the femur
(B) Abnormal lateral rotation during extension
(C) Abnormal passive abduction of the extended leg
(D) Inability to lock the knee on full extension

61. Which one of the following conditions would result in a negative nitrogen balance?

(A) Consumption of dietary proteins that are deficient in glycine
(B) Normal intake of dietary protein accompanied by defective cholecystokinin-pancreozymin (CCK-PZ) production
(C) Nitrogen consumption that exceeds nitrogen excretion
(D) A tyrosine supplement in the diet of a child with phenylketonuria
(E) A 50% reduction in the hydrochloric acid (HCl) content of gastric juice

62. A young child develops pharyngitis, a fever, and a rash. β-Hemolytic, gram-positive cocci in chains are isolated from the throat and are found to be catalase-negative. All of the following statements about the virulence factors of this pathogen are true EXCEPT

(A) hemolysis results from production of extracellular hemolysins
(B) the organism produces M protein, which has antiphagocytic properties
(C) The organism produces lipoteichoic acid, which is necessary for attachment to mucosa
(D) the organism is not encapsulated
(E) the rash is produced by a toxin distinct from the hemolysins

63. A patient hospitalized for multiple fractures was placed on a prophylactic antibiotic. Two days prior to discharge, diarrhea developed requiring intravenous rehydration. The antibiotic was changed to a broad-spectrum cephalosporin, but diarrhea continued and the patient's condition deteriorated. All of the following actions are appropriate EXCEPT

(A) sigmoidoscopic examination
(B) proper isolation of the patient
(C) Gram stain of feces for white blood cells
(D) a request for *Clostridium difficile* toxin test
(E) changing the antibiotic to clindamycin

64. A 5-year-old child in Bangladesh drinks untreated river water and develops cholera. Which of the following scenarios is most likely to occur?

(A) Recovery following treatment is slow because *Vibrio cholerae* causes chronic intracellular infections
(B) Microscopic examination of stools reveals leukocytes
(C) Disease symptoms arise due to enterotoxin inhibition of protein synthesis in intestinal cells
(D) *V. cholerae* attaches to the intestinal mucosa

65. Surgical instruments are boiled for 10 minutes in a saline solution containing *Escherichia coli, Mycobacterium tuberculosis,* and *Bacillus cereus*. What outcome of those listed can be expected?

(A) *E. coli* will survive this boiling because it has a thick peptidoglycan cell wall
(B) *M. tuberculosis* will survive this boiling because of its waxy cell wall
(C) *B. cereus* will survive this boiling because it is a spore-former

66. Cushing's syndrome is a complex array of symptoms due to excess glucocorticoid activity. All of the following statements about Cushing's syndrome are correct EXCEPT

(A) the disease may be associated with an adenoma of the pituitary corticotropes
(B) the disease may be secondary to abnormal hypothalamic function with excessive release of corticotropin releasing factor (CRF)
(C) the disease may be due to ectopic adrenocorticotropic hormone (ACTH) synthesis
(D) some aspects of the syndrome may be due to long-standing administration of glucocorticoids
(E) injection of 1 mg of dexamethasone reduces cortisol levels in a normal subject to 5 µg/dl and in a patient with Cushing's syndrome to less than detectable levels

Questions 67–73

A 27-year-old man who has torn his anterior cruciate ligament (ACL) while skiing is sent to the operating room for ACL replacement and reconstruction. The anesthesiologist selects halothane.

67. Important adverse effects of halothane include all of the following EXCEPT

(A) depression of respiratory drive
(B) lowering of ventilatory response to CO_2
(C) malignant hyperthermia in genetically sensitive individuals
(D) lowering of the seizure threshold
(E) depressed myocardial contractility

68. Induction of anesthesia is smooth, and the operation begins. Before an incision is made in the subclavian region, the surgical resident informs the surgeon that this surgery is to be performed on the

(A) ankle
(B) knee
(C) hip
(D) elbow
(E) shoulder

69. The ACL stabilizes this joint by attaching the

(A) medial malleolus of the tibia to the talus
(B) lateral malleolus of the fibula to the talus
(C) head of the femur to the innominate (hip) bone
(D) femur to the fibula
(E) femur to the tibia

70. The head of the femur is attached to the innominate bone at the cup-shaped region known as the

(A) ilioischial fossa
(B) iliofemoral fossa
(C) ischial depression
(D) acetabulum
(E) sella turcica

71. Most long bone growth occurs at the

(A) epiphysis
(B) diaphysis
(C) epiphyseal plate
(D) medullary cavity
(E) primary ossification center

72. All of the following bones are carpal bones EXCEPT

(A) capitate
(B) cuboid
(C) navicular
(D) trapezium
(E) trapezoid

73. The fundamental unit of compact bone is the

(A) haversian system
(B) osteoblast–osteoclast dyad
(C) canaliculus
(D) osteocyte
(E) calcium hydroxyapatite

74. The inhibition observed in the Lineweaver-Burk plot below is subject to which one of the following actions? It

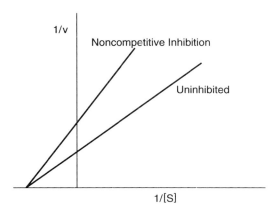

(A) can be reversed by a high concentration of substrate
(B) results from compounds that are transition-state analogs
(C) occurs through the interaction of the inhibitor at the active site
(D) results in a decrease in the V_{max} of the reaction
(E) is characterized by an increase in the K_m for the substrate

75. In humans, the major route of nitrogen metabolism from amino acids to urea involves which one of the following sets of enzymes?

(A) Amino acid oxidases and arginase
(B) Glutaminase and amino acid oxidases
(C) Glutamate dehydrogenase and transaminases
(D) Transaminases and glutaminase
(E) Glutamine synthetase and urease

76. All of the following statements about allosteric enzymes are true EXCEPT

(A) positive cooperativity sensitizes the enzyme to small changes in substrate concentration
(B) they frequently catalyze the slowest step in a metabolic pathway
(C) they are composed of subunits that may be either identical or nonidentical
(D) the binding of a ligand to the allosteric site induces a conformational change in the activity site
(E) they have substrate saturation curves that are described by Michaelis-Menten kinetics

77. Major risk factors for the development of chronic obstructive pulmonary disease (COPD) include all of the following EXCEPT

(A) smoking
(B) air pollution
(C) occupational exposure to irritant gases and particles
(D) α_1-antitrypsin deficiency
(E) intravenous drug abuse

78. Captopril is useful in the treatment of systemic hypertension because it

(A) blocks the effect of angiotensin II at its receptor in the central nervous system (CNS)
(B) directly relaxes vascular smooth muscle
(C) inhibits the movement of extracellular calcium into myocardial cells
(D) decreases the activity of angiotensin-converting enzyme
(E) inhibits the production of renin

79. Tamoxifen can control the growth of some forms of female breast cancer by

(A) inhibiting estrogen synthesis
(B) inhibiting estrogen-induced DNA transcription
(C) competing for estrogen receptors
(D) inhibiting the secretion of luteinizing hormone (LH)
(E) stimulating nuclear transcription

80. Which of the following statements most accurately describes specific features of neuromuscular transmission?

(A) Each muscle fiber contains multiple axon terminals
(B) The end-plate is highly enriched in electrically excitable gates
(C) Enzymatic degradation of the transmitter can terminate transmission
(D) Acetylcholine (ACh) causes Na^+ channels to open as a result of membrane depolarization

Questions 81 and 82

A patient weighing 50 kg is given a 20 mg/kg dose of a new drug. The plasma concentrations determined over time are illustrated in the graph below.

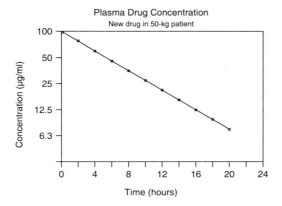

81. The drug's volume of distribution (V_d) is approximately

(A) 200 ml
(B) 1 L
(C) 2 L
(D) 10 L
(E) insufficient information to answer

82. The half-life of elimination of this drug was approximately

(A) 1 hour
(B) 4 hours
(C) 6 hours
(D) 10 hours
(E) insufficient information to answer

83. True statements about the side chains of amino acids that are found in proteins include which one of the following?

(A) Glutamine provides strong buffering capacity of pH 7.0
(B) Lysine absorbs ultraviolet light
(C) Glutamic acid and aspartic acid have an isoelectric pH (pI)
(D) Proline terminates α-helical regions
(E) Only D-amino acids are incorporated into protein

84. A previously healthy 27-year-old woman is seen because of a petechial rash. She denies any recent bleeding and has had no recent illnesses. Hemoglobin, hematocrit, and white blood cell counts are normal. Examination of the peripheral blood smear reveals normal red and white blood cells and is remarkable only for a paucity of platelets. The most likely diagnosis in this patient is

(A) aleukemic leukemia
(B) idiopathic thrombocytopenic purpura (ITP)
(C) Glanzmann's thrombasthenia
(D) amegakaryocytic thrombocytopenia
(E) drug-induced thrombocytopenia

85. A 55-year-old man with a history of chronic alcoholism presents with complaints of fatigue and weakness. His laboratory values are as follows:

Hgb/Hct	11.5/34.0	
MCV	110	
MCH	38.0	
RDW	19.5	
WBC	$6.0 \times 10^9/L$	
Differential:		
Polys	80%	$4.8 \times 10^9/L$
Bands	7%	$0.42 \times 10^9/L$
Lymphs	10%	$0.6 \times 10^9/L$
Monos	5%	$0.3 \times 10^9/L$

Microscopic examination of a peripheral blood smear shows poikilocytosis and hypersegmented neutrophils. This patient is most likely to have

(A) anemia due to folate or vitamin B_{12} deficiency
(B) anemia due to iron deficiency
(C) anemia following hemorrhage
(D) sickle cell anemia
(E) thalassemia minor

86. All of the following statements about RNA are correct EXCEPT

(A) an mRNA molecule is translated once and is then degraded
(B) ribosomal RNA is formed by transcription of a family of repeated nuclear genes
(C) the ribosome, which is a complex of RNA and protein, is the site of protein synthesis
(D) three different RNA polymerase enzymes are required for sustained protein synthesis in human cells
(E) tRNA molecules contain an anticodon loop that pairs with the triplet codon of mRNA

87. In which region of the human respiratory system are Clara cells primarily found?

(A) Trachea
(B) Extrapulmonary bronchi
(C) Nasopharyngeal cavity
(D) Bronchioles
(E) Alveoli

88. Of the following statements about mRNA production, the most accurate is that it

(A) proceeds by synthesis of the RNA in the 3' to 5' direction
(B) involves the removal of internal regions of DNA from the genome
(C) occurs exclusively in the cytoplasm of the human cell
(D) may be regulated by hormones
(E) involves the post-transcriptional addition of adenylate nucleotides to the 5' end of the molecule

89. Stimulation by glucose of the beta cells of the islets of Langerhans of the endocrine pancreas causes

(A) enhancement of gluconeogenesis in the liver
(B) increased glycogenolysis by the liver
(C) stimulation of the release of glucagon
(D) increased synthesis of triglycerides and fatty acids in adipose tissue
(E) decreased oxidation of amino acids in the liver

90. The most important allosteric activator of glycolysis in the liver is which one of the following compounds?

(A) Fructose 2,6-bisphosphate
(B) Acetylcoenzyme A (acetyl CoA)
(C) Adenosine triphosphate (ATP)
(D) Citrate
(E) Glucose 6-phosphate

91. A rational approach for the treatment of ventricular tachycardia associated with myocardial ischemia in a hospitalized patient includes the use of

(A) digitalis
(B) diltiazem
(C) lidocaine
(D) propranolol
(E) verapamil

92. If end diastolic volume is approximately 115 ml in the volume–pressure curve of the left ventricle below, then which of the following statements is most accurate?

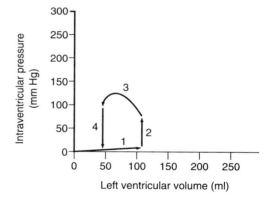

(A) The ejection fraction is approximately 30%
(B) Aortic diastolic pressure is approximately 80 mm Hg
(C) Isovolumic contraction is during the section labeled 3
(D) Stroke volume is approximately 45 ml
(E) Left ventricular end diastolic pressure is approximately 100 mm Hg

93. Each of the following structures refers pain to the inguinal region along the lumbar splanchnic nerves EXCEPT the

(A) kidneys
(B) bladder
(C) sigmoid colon
(D) descending colon
(E) uterus

94. Capsule production is essential for the virulence of many pathogenic bacteria. Which of the following statements best describes bacterial capsules?

(A) The most important function of the *Streptococcus pneumoniae* capsule is adhesion
(B) The capsule of *Hemophilus influenzae* type B stimulates T-cell–dependent immune response
(C) Opsonizing antibodies are often directed against *Streptococcus pneumoniae* capsules
(D) The capsule of group B *Neisseria meningitidis* is protein
(E) The DPT vaccine currently licensed contains purified *Bordetella pertussis* capsules

95. Triglycerides are neutral fats of animals and food plants; they make up about 90% of the dietary intake of fats. An important step in their digestive fate in the gastrointestinal tract is

(A) significant hydrolysis by gastric lipases
(B) breakdown by biliary enzymes
(C) formation of fatty acids and monoglyceride by pancreatic lipase
(D) active transport of fatty acid products in the intestinal brush border

96. The pressor response to an indirect-acting sympathomimetic agent, such as amphetamine, is

(A) associated with marked tolerance (tachyphylaxis)
(B) decreased in the presence of a monoamine oxidase (MAO) inhibitor
(C) potentiated by an uptake 1 inhibitor, such as imipramine
(D) potentiated by pretreatment with reserpine
(E) related to its direct effects on postsynaptic receptors

97. If an individual had a genetic defect in the enzyme that produces N-acetylglutamate, the most likely clinical finding would be hyperammonemia with

(A) elevated levels of argininosuccinate (the condensation product of citrulline and aspartate)
(B) no detectable citrulline
(C) elevated levels of arginine
(D) elevated levels of urea
(E) no detectable ornithine

98. The extraction of β-hydroxybutyrate from blood and its oxidation to CO_2 and H_2O requires the participation of

(A) β-hydroxybutyrate dehydrogenase and hydroxymethylglutaryl coenzyme A (HMG CoA) lyase
(B) acetoacetate thiokinase and β-hydroxybutyrate dehydrogenase
(C) HMG CoA synthase and thiolase
(D) short-chain fatty acyl CoA dehydrogenase and thiolase
(E) succinyl CoA: acetoacetate acyltransferase and HMG CoA lyase

99. At which of these blood neutrophil levels do patients acquire a significant risk of opportunistic infection?

(A) < $1000/\mu l$
(B) 1000 to $1500/\mu l$
(C) 1500 to $2000/\mu l$
(D) 2000 to $2500/\mu l$
(E) 2500 to $3000/\mu l$

100. Restriction enzymes have which one of the following characteristics? They

(A) can only cleave circular DNA
(B) generate either staggered (sticky) or blunt ends upon cleaving DNA
(C) cleave different DNAs randomly
(D) can cleave different DNAs only once
(E) can cleave both DNA and RNA

101. Characteristics of Duchenne muscular dystrophy (DMD) include all of the following EXCEPT

(A) decreased amounts of dystrophin in affected muscles
(B) hypertrophy of affected muscle groups
(C) autosomal dominant inheritance via mutated chromosome 19
(D) one-third of the cases resulting from spontaneous mutation
(E) sarcomere hypercontraction and contraction band formation

102. What condition is marked by formation of a malignant pustule?

(A) Enteritis necroticans
(B) Lockjaw
(C) Cutaneous anthrax
(D) Pseudomembranous colitis
(E) Woolsorter's disease

103. Of the following amino acids, which one is released from skeletal muscle in amounts that exceed its relative abundance in muscle protein?

(A) Aspartate
(B) Alanine
(C) Glutamate
(D) Leucine
(E) Tyrosine

104. The graph below measures the number of viable bacterial cells in a control culture and cultures of exponentially growing cells to which antibiotics were added at the point indicated by the arrow. The antibiotic added to the culture to produce curve A was which one of the following?

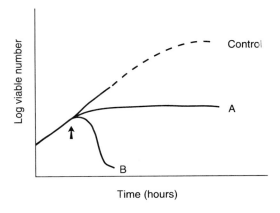

(A) Polymyxin B
(B) Cephalothin
(C) Chloramphenicol
(D) Methicillin
(E) Vancomycin

105. The plasma membrane is composed of lipids and proteins with the basic structure of a lipid bilayer. Correct statements regarding the structure and function of the plasma membrane include all of the following EXCEPT

(A) phospholipids are amphipathic
(B) proteins may penetrate either portion of or the entire bilayer
(C) phospholipids promote free diffusion of ions and small watersoluble molecules
(D) proteins are amphipathic
(E) some large proteins are free to diffuse laterally in the plane of the membrane

Questions 106 and 107

A 68-year-old woman suddenly develops a fever of 38.2° C and a severe headache one evening. The following morning she also experiences a stiff neck and uncharacteristic drowsiness. At the emergency room, her temperature is 38.8° C, and there is pain and resistance on flexion of her neck. The patient is noted to be mentally competent although lethargic. A cerebral spinal fluid (CSF) sample is obtained by lumbar puncture.

106. On the basis of the history and physical examination of this patient, what is the most probable diagnosis?

(A) Viral meningitis
(B) Fungal meningitis
(C) Bacterial meningitis
(D) Viral encephalitis
(E) Brain abscess

107. On the basis of the patient's age, the probable etiologic agent is

(A) *Staphylococcus aureus*
(B) *Hemophilus influenzae*
(C) *Streptococcus pneumoniae*
(D) *Neisseria meningitidis*
(E) none of the above

108. Cholesterol biosynthesis occurs in the cytosol of many cells of the body, primarily in the liver, and entails all of the following steps EXCEPT it

(A) forms lanosterol from squalene and then converts it to cholesterol
(B) requires NADPH as a source of reducing equivalents
(C) forms β-hydroxy-β-methylglutaryl coenzyme A (HMG CoA) from acetoacetyl CoA
(D) forms squalene from isoprenoid units
(E) uses HMG CoA reductase for catalysis of HMG CoA to mevinolin

109. Each statement below concerning the contraction of myofibrils in skeletal muscle is true EXCEPT

(A) the size of the A band decreases
(B) the size of the H band decreases
(C) the size of the I band decreases
(D) thin filaments penetrate the A band
(E) Z disks are drawn closer to the A band

110. Ingestion of 150 mEq of Na^+/day is usually balanced by excretion of a similar amount in urine. Since glomerular filtration normally contains 26,000 mEq of Na^+/day, several important Na^+ reabsorbing mechanisms have evolved, including all of the following EXCEPT

(A) active transport of Na^+ from inside proximal epithelial cells to interstitial spaces
(B) passive cotransport of Na^+ with glucose or amino acids in the proximal tubular epithelium
(C) active transport in the thick segment of the loop of Henle
(D) hormone-independent passive reabsorption in the distal tubular epithelium

111. The most important prognostic factor for human cancer is

(A) tumor grade
(B) tumor stage
(C) lymphocytic infiltration
(D) vascular invasion
(E) the mitotic index

112. Which of the following proteins is penicillin-binding?

(A) Alanine racemase
(B) Glycine pentapeptide
(C) Peptidoglycan
(D) Porin protein
(E) Transpeptidase

113. Enteric pathogens vary with respect to their ability to invade the intestinal mucosa. After infection, which one of the intestinal pathogens listed is most likely to invade the intestinal tract and then spread throughout the body?

(A) *Vibrio cholerae*
(B) *Salmonella typhi*
(C) *Shigella dysenteriae*
(D) Nontyphoid *Salmonella*
(E) *Campylobacter jejuni*

114. For antibiotic therapy, it is useful to understand both the action of the prescribed antibiotic and the pathogenesis of the bacteria responsible for a patient's infection. For example, the aminoglycoside antibiotic gentamicin does not enter mammalian cells and therefore is ineffective against intracellular pathogens. Considering only this information, gentamicin is effective against all of the following infections EXCEPT

(A) *Hemophilus influenzae* type B epiglottitis
(B) *Pseudomonas aeruginosa* burn infections
(C) *Klebsiella pneumoniae* respiratory infections
(D) *Escherichia coli* urinary tract infections
(E) *Salmonella typhi* enteric fevers

115. Hepatic gluconeogenesis from alanine requires the participation of

(A) glucose 6-phosphatase and pyruvate kinase
(B) phosphofructokinase and pyruvate carboxylase
(C) pyruvate carboxylase and phosphoenolpyruvate carboxykinase (PEPCK)
(D) fructose 1,6-diphosphatase and pyruvate kinase
(E) transaminase and phosphofructokinase

116. Tricyclic antidepressants (e.g., imipramine and amitriptyline) are useful agents for the management of endogenous depression because they

(A) reverse symptoms within days after administration
(B) have little effect on cardiovascular function
(C) affect only dopamine receptors within the central nervous system (CNS)
(D) affect neuronal amine uptake mechanisms
(E) deplete brain serotonin levels

117. RNA processing can be best described by which of the following statements? It

(A) occurs in the cytoplasm
(B) results in the addition of nucleotides to the primary transcript of ribosomal RNA
(C) results in the formation of new covalent bonds between RNA and DNA
(D) includes the addition of a tail of polyadenylic acid at the 5' end
(E) includes the methylation of nucleotides in RNA

118. All of the following statements about protein synthesis are true EXCEPT

(A) the activated form of an amino acid is called aminoacyl tRNA
(B) the only energy required is for the synthesis of aminoacyl tRNA
(C) the formation of the peptide bond is catalyzed by peptidyltransferase
(D) synthesis occurs in the mitochondria as well as in the cytoplasm of cells
(E) synthesis does not occur in the absence of RNA

119. Translation of a synthetic polyribonucleotide containing the repeating sequence CAA in a cell-free protein synthesizing system produced three homopolypeptides: polyglutamine, polyasparagine, and polythreonine. If the codons for glutamine and asparagine are CAA and AAC, respectively, which of the following triplets is a codon for threonine?

(A) AAC
(B) CAA
(C) CAC
(D) CCA
(E) ACA

120. A 38-year-old man with AIDS develops meningitis. Microscopic examination of his spinal fluid shows yeast cells. India ink staining of these yeasts shows a visible clear halo surrounding each cell. Which one of the following pathogens is responsible for the man's meningitis?

(A) A virus
(B) *Cryptococcus neoformans*
(C) *Hemophilus influenzae*
(D) *Neisseria meningitidis*
(E) *Candida albicans*

121. Resistance to phagocytosis is among the most important properties for virulence of many bacteria. *Mycobacterium tuberculosis* is very resistant to phagocytic killing and actually grows in macrophages. The successful antiphagocytic strategy employed by *M. tuberculosis* clearly involves which one of the following mechanisms?

(A) Production of protein exotoxins to kill or impair the phagocyte
(B) Prevention of phagosome–lysosome fusion
(C) Elaboration of IgA protease
(D) Production of an antiphagocytic polysaccharide capsule
(E) Escape from the phagolysosome into the cytoplasm

Questions 122–129

A 27-year-old woman presents with muscle weakness, including eyelid ptosis, slurred speech, and difficulty swallowing. The history reveals that the woman is being treated for a gram-negative infection with gentamicin. The following tests have been ordered: thyroid function studies, serum creatine kinase, an electromyogram, and a muscle biopsy.

122. The attending physician chides the resident on the case for not ordering edrophonium, which produces a dramatic improvement in the patient's muscle strength when administered intravenously. All of the other tests that were ordered returned with normal values. The resident's working diagnosis is

(A) Duchenne muscular dystrophy (DMD)
(B) monoadenylate deaminase deficiency
(C) myasthenia gravis
(D) hyperthyroidism
(E) toxic drug myopathy

123. This patient's condition most likely results from

(A) inadequate acetylcholinesterase in the synaptic cleft
(B) production of defective acetylcholine (ACh) receptors
(C) impaired synthesis or storage of ACh in presynaptic vesicles
(D) impaired release of ACh from presynaptic terminals
(E) blockade and increased turnover of ACh receptors

124. Aminoglycoside antibiotics create and exacerbate muscle weakness through

(A) inhibition of presynaptic release of ACh
(B) antagonism of the action of acetylcholinesterase
(C) potentiation of the action of acetylcholinesterase
(D) increasing the turnover of ACh receptors
(E) slowing conduction of the action potential

125. The adverse effects of the aminoglycoside antibiotics can be overcome with the intravenous administration of

(A) magnesium gluconate
(B) calcium gluconate
(C) magnesium phosphate
(D) calcium citrate
(E) creatine phosphate

126. Besides the aminoglycosides, another drug known to create muscle weakness is

(A) puromycin
(B) actinomycin
(C) tetracycline
(D) penicillamine
(E) amoxicillin

127. A more thorough physical examination of this patient would likely reveal an abnormal

(A) adrenal
(B) heart
(C) kidney
(D) thymus
(E) thyroid

128. Primary treatment of this patient's condition should begin with

(A) isoflurophate (di*iso*propyl phosphorofluoridate; DFP)
(B) mefenamic acid
(C) pralidoxime
(D) pyridostigmine
(E) triorthocresylphosphate

129. Long-term treatment should also include

(A) echothiophate
(B) edrophonium
(C) glucocorticoids
(D) pralidoxime
(E) vitamin and mineral supplementation

130. Which one of the following factors differentiates viruses from *Chlamydia*?

(A) Obligate intracellular parasitism
(B) The need for arthropod vectors
(C) Dependency on the host cell for energy
(D) The presence of a single type of nucleic acid

131. Which one of the following drugs or chemicals has been associated with the induction of aplastic anemia?

(A) Acetaminophen
(B) Methyldopa
(C) Benzene
(D) Penicillin
(E) Thiouracil

Questions 132–137

A 50-year-old man presents to the emergency room with severe epigastric pain, low-grade fever, tachycardia, and mild hypotension. The patient relates a history of moderate to heavy social drinking. The chief resident suspects acute pancreatitis.

132. The single most important laboratory finding to confirm the diagnosis of pancreatitis would be

(A) hyperlipidemia
(B) hyperbilirubinemia
(C) elevated serum amylase
(D) elevated serum phospholipase A
(E) elevated serum alkaline phosphatase

133. Which of the following polypeptide hormones is stimulated by increased acid from the stomach and subsequently stimulates the release of pancreatic juice rich in electrolytes and water?

(A) Gastrin
(B) Secretin
(C) Cholecystokinin
(D) Pancreozymin
(E) Vasoactive intestinal polypeptide (VIP)

134. Which of the following hormones is produced by the duodenal and upper jejunal mucosa and stimulates the release of pancreatic juice rich in digestive enzymes?

(A) Cholecystokinin
(B) Secretin
(C) Glucagon
(D) Pancreatic polypeptide
(E) VIP

135. Neuronal control of pancreatic exocrine function is mediated by

(A) VIP
(B) dopamine
(C) serotonin
(D) substance P
(E) acetylcholine (ACh)

136. The hormones secretin and cholecystokinin promote their actions on the pancreas via the

(A) hepatic portal system
(B) pancreatic duct
(C) common bile duct
(D) lymphatics
(E) bloodstream

137. The principal reason that the pancreas does not autodigest is that

(A) proteolytic enzymes are secreted as proenzymes
(B) pancreatic acini and ducts secrete a protective mucopolysaccharide, which lines their walls
(C) the pancreas maintains a slightly alkaline pH, rendering the digestive enzymes inactive
(D) pancreatic parenchyma is high in hydroxyproline, which is resistant to proteolysis
(E) proper enzyme substrates are not present

138. Low levels of cellular β-hydroxy-β-methylglutaryl coenzyme A (HMG CoA) reductase activity in humans is most likely to result from

(A) a vegetarian diet
(B) the administration of a bile acid sequestering resin
(C) familial hypercholesterolemia
(D) a long-term high cholesterol diet

139. *Pseudomonas aeruginosa, Staphylococcus aureus,* and *Serratia marcescens* produce which one of the following compounds?

(A) Endotoxins
(B) Enterotoxins
(C) Lipoteichoic acids
(D) Mycolic acids
(E) Pigments

Questions 140 and 141

The left ventricular and aortic pressure tracings below were recorded during cardiac catheterization of a 62-year-old patient who complains of chest pain and dizziness on exertion.

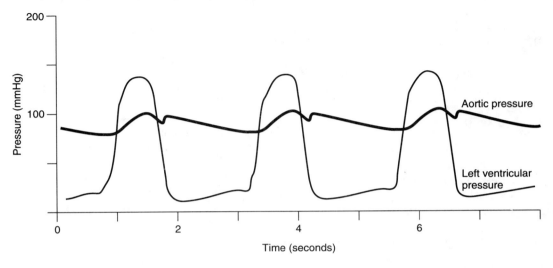

140. The left ventricular and aortic pressure tracings indicate that this patient has

(A) pulmonary stenosis
(B) aortic stenosis
(C) mitral stenosis
(D) aortic insufficiency
(E) mitral insufficiency

141. The most likely change in heart sound in this patient would be

(A) systolic murmur
(B) diastolic murmur
(C) presystolic murmur
(D) mid-diastolic murmur

142. Which of the following statements best describes the genetic code? It

(A) varies considerably from one organism to another
(B) is composed of codewords containing three nucleotide letters
(C) represents all of the nucleotide sequence information within a transcription unit
(D) contains start and stop signals for specific terminating amino acids
(E) contains only one codeword for each amino acid

143. Cimetidine and ranitidine are examples of antihistamines that

(A) cause sedation
(B) are useful for motion sickness
(C) enhance hepatic drug-metabolizing enzymes
(D) reduce gastric acid secretion
(E) are useful in the treatment of certain allergies

144. All of the following statements about collagen formation are true EXCEPT

(A) hydroxylation of proline requires molecular oxygen and α-ketoglutarate
(B) the triple helix forms after removal of the globular ends
(C) glycosylation occurs prior to hydroxylation
(D) assembly of tropocollagen into collagen fibrils is necessary for secretion
(E) the stability of the triple helix decreases with increasing hydroxyproline content

145. Which of the statements below concerning the disaccharide pictured is most accurate? It

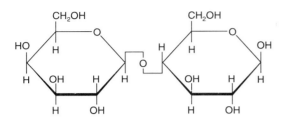

(A) yields a negative result in the Fehling-Benedict reducing sugar test
(B) is cleaved by isomaltose
(C) is a β-galactoside
(D) is digested and absorbed by a lactase-deficient child
(E) is a good source of calories for a 2-week-old child with galactosemia

146. Chronic type B (antral) gastritis is characterized by all of the following features EXCEPT

(A) glandular atrophy with the presence of very few short, cystically dilated glands
(B) circulating antibodies to parietal cells and intrinsic factor
(C) excess acid secretion with low intragastric pH and, frequently, duodenal ulcers
(D) low serum gastrin levels
(E) flattened or absent rugal folds

147. The S_3 heart sound is normally heard only in children or young, thin-chested adults. An accentuated S_3 heart sound can sometimes be heard in either children or adults with all of the following pathologies EXCEPT

(A) mitral regurgitation
(B) patent ductus arteriosus
(C) left ventricular failure
(D) pulmonary stenosis
(E) ventricular septal defects

148. Which of the following statements concerning primitive aortic arches and their derivatives is true?

(A) The left fourth aortic arch forms the arch of the aorta
(B) The right sixth aortic arch forms the right subclavian artery
(C) The left fifth aortic arch forms the ductus arteriosus
(D) The first aortic arch forms the common carotid artery

149. Phenytoin (Dilantin) is effective in most forms of epilepsy (with the exception of absence seizures) because it

(A) directly binds to chloride channels in the central nervous system (CNS)
(B) enhances the inhibitory actions of gamma-aminobutyrate (GABA) at its receptor in the CNS
(C) affects Na^+ conductance in neurons via voltage-sensitive Na^+-channel inhibition
(D) is usually started concurrently with phenobarbital therapy

150. According to Fick's law, O_2 consumption is equal to the product of blood flow and arteriovenous oxygen difference. If the lungs absorb 300 ml/min of oxygen, arterial oxygen content is 20 ml/100 ml blood, pulmonary arterial oxygen content is 15 ml/100 ml blood, and heart rate is 60/min, then stroke volume is

(A) 50 ml
(B) 60 ml
(C) 100 ml
(D) 5 L/min
(E) 6 L/min

151. In the figure below, the oxyhemoglobin dissociation curve is shown for a normal patient and for an anemic patient. A true statement concerning these patients is which one of the following?

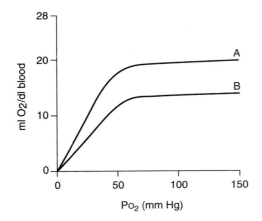

(A) Patient A is anemic
(B) Arterial P_{O_2} is identical for both subjects
(C) Venous P_{O_2} of the anemic subject will be greater than that of the normal subject at rest or during exercise
(D) If cardiac output is identical, then oxygen delivery will be identical in subjects A and B

152. Pathogenic bacteria enter the body by various routes, and entry mechanisms are critical for understanding the pathogenesis and transmissibility of each agent. Which one of the following is a correct association between a pathogen and its common entry mechanism?

(A) *Neisseria meningitidis*—sexually transmitted entry
(B) *Corynebacterium diphtheriae* — food-borne entry
(C) *Rickettsia rickettsii*—entry by contamination of wound with soil
(D) *Clostridium tetani*—inhalation entry
(E) *Borrelia burgdorferi*—arthropod vector–borne entry

153. A monoclonal antibody that neutralizes endotoxin has been produced. This antibody has tremendous therapeutic potential for patients suffering septic shock from endotoxemia. This antibody would be useful in treating patients with bacteremia caused by all of the following organisms EXCEPT

(A) *Proteus vulgaris*
(B) *Bacillus anthracis*
(C) *Escherichia coli*
(D) *Klebsiella pneumoniae*
(E) *Serratia marcescens*

154. If forbidden clones are not deleted during T-cell development, a person may develop

(A) hypogammaglobulinemia
(B) a type I hypersensitivity reaction to exogenous antigens
(C) an autoimmune disease
(D) tolerance to autoantigens

155. Which one of the following fatty acids is always required in the diet of humans?

(A) Linoleic acid
(B) Phytanic acid
(C) Arachidonic acid
(D) Palmitic acid
(E) Decanoic acid

156. All of the following statements about enzymes are true EXCEPT that

(A) V_{max} is a measure of catalytic efficiency
(B) K_m is a measure of the enzyme's affinity for the substrate
(C) formation of the substrate complex results in rearrangement of specific functional groups of the enzyme
(D) the reaction rate is accelerated by increasing the energy of the transition state
(E) they frequently use ionizable amino acid side chains as general acids and bases in catalysis

157. Type II pneumocytes have all of the following characteristics EXCEPT

(A) they elaborate pulmonary surfactant
(B) they exhibit surface microvilli
(C) they make up most of the alveolar surface area
(D) they contain osmiophilic lamellar bodies
(E) defects in these cells contribute to infant and adult respiratory distress

158. A 2-year-old child is hospitalized with splenomegaly, anemia, hypersplenism, and hepatomegaly. Enzyme studies show a deficiency of lysosomal β-galactosidase activity and an absence of glucocerebrosidase with an accumulation of β-glucosylceramide in macrophages and hepatocytes. The lipid storage disease most likely to be diagnosed in this child is

(A) Niemann-Pick disease
(B) Gaucher's disease
(C) Gangliosidosis
(D) Tay-Sachs disease

159. Each condition below is associated with an increased incidence of endometrial carcinoma EXCEPT

(A) obesity
(B) diabetes
(C) use of oral contraceptives
(D) hypertension
(E) infertility

160. Volume and pressure (alveolar, P_A; pleural, P_{PL}) for a normal respiratory cycle are shown in the figure below. Correct statements about respiration include which one of the following?

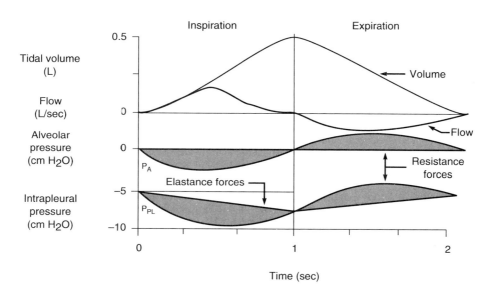

(A) Inspiration is the result of a passive process
(B) Gas flow is greatest at the end of inspiration
(C) Elastic recoil of the lung is identical at the beginning and end of inspiration
(D) During expiration, alveolar pressure becomes greater than atmospheric pressure

Directions: Each group of items in this section consists of lettered options followed by a set of numbered items. For each item, select the **one** lettered option that is most closely associated with it. Each lettered option may be selected once, more than once, or not at all.

Questions 161–165

For each characteristic of a vitamin deficiency listed below, select the disease with which it is most likely to be associated.

(A) Pellagra
(B) Beriberi
(C) Both
(D) Neither

161. Results from a nicotinic acid (niacin) deficiency

162. Results from a thiamine hydrochloride (vitamin B_1) deficiency

163. Results from a riboflavin (vitamin B_2) deficiency

164. Presents with diarrhea and dermatitis

165. Progresses to degenerative changes in the central nervous system (CNS)

Questions 166–170

Match each of the following conditions with the appropriate syndrome.

(A) Sheehan's syndrome
(B) Cushing's syndrome
(C) Conn's syndrome
(D) Waterhouse-Friderichsen syndrome
(E) Bartter's syndrome

166. Hyperreninemia

167. Anterior pituitary infarction

168. An overproduction of cortisol

169. Widespread petechiae, purpura, or hemorrhages

170. Aldosterone-producing adenoma

Questions 171–175

For each artery or vein comprising the vasculature of the cranium, select the lettered foramen or fissure through which it courses, shown on the illustration of the inferior aspect of the cranium below.

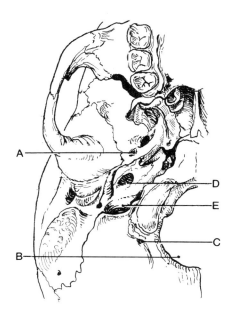

171. Middle meningeal artery

172. Internal carotid artery

173. Internal jugular vein

174. Emissary vein

175. Vertebral artery

Questions 176–180

Match the pulse and pressure readings listed below with the most likely diagnosis.

	Age	Sex	Pulse, supine	Blood pressure, supine	Pulse, sitting	Blood pressure, sitting
176.	74	F	60	140/80	65	128/85
177.	59	M	62	140/80	85	135/75
178.	68	M	72	138/76	74	124/63
179.	81	F	88	154/86	92	150/88
180.	63	M	64	145/92	66	147/94

(A) Normal
(B) Isolated systolic hypertension
(C) Autonomic neuropathy (e.g., diabetic neuropathy)
(D) Hypovolemia (dehydration)
(E) Hypertension

Questions 181–185

For each lipoprotein type listed below, select the genetic disorder that is most likely to be associated with it.

(A) Combined hyperlipidemia
(B) Hypertriglyceridemia
(C) Type III hyperlipoproteinemia
(D) Hypercholesterolemia
(E) Lipoprotein lipase deficiency

181. Chylomicrons

182. Low-density lipoproteins (LDL)

183. Chylomicron remnants and intermediate-density lipoproteins

184. Very low-density lipoproteins (VLDL)

185. VLDL and chylomicrons

Questions 186–191

Lung tumors can at times have similar gross and microscopic appearances, but generally distinguishing features can be observed for the major tumor classes. Match the following descriptive features of malignant tumors with the correct neoplasm.

(A) Squamous cell carcinoma
(B) Adenocarcinoma (usual type)
(C) Adenocarcinoma (bronchioalveolar type)
(D) Large cell carcinoma
(E) Small cell (oat cell) carcinoma
(F) Carcinoid

186. Centrally located in major airways near the hilum; may have endobronchial element; large cells with optically dense cytoplasm form large irregular sheets with central necrosis; intercellular bridges; prominent host response; hypercalcemia

187. Grows along alveolar septa; multicentric foci; cuboidal or columnar cells with abundant mucus production; huge nuclei with almost no cytoplasm

188. Peripherally located; often associated with a preexisting scar; glandular, mucinous, or papillary growth pattern; prominent nucleoli; most likely to produce hypertrophic osteoarthropathy

189. Often protrudes into the bronchus like a polyp; highly vascularized; small cells with monotonous round or fusiform nuclei; 80- to 250-nm neurosecretory granules; often benign, with a 10-year survival rate of approximately 50%

190. Usually peripherally located; grows in sheets with areas of necrosis; small cells with scant cytoplasm and nucleoli that are not prominent; dense 80- to 140-nm neurosecretory granules; poor survival due to extensive metastases

191. Grows in sheets or in large gland-like structures with dense stroma; large cells (30 μm to 50 μm) with pale cytoplasm; oval nuclei with prominent nucleoli; leukemoid reaction; polymorphonuclear infiltrates; extensive local spread with metastasis often to the brain

Questions 192–194

Match each description below with the appropriate lettered structure in this scanning electron micrograph of liver parenchymal tissue.

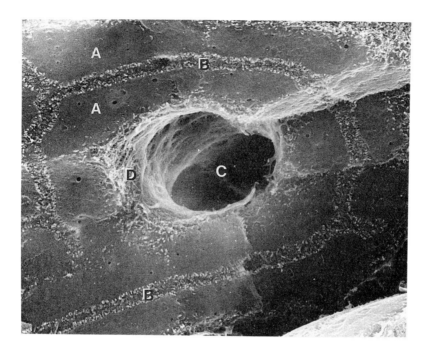

192. Receives blood from the portal vein and hepatic artery and drains blood into the central vein

193. A liver parenchymal cell

194. A bile canaliculus surrounded by tight junctions that form the blood–bile barrier

Questions 195–199

Match the physical manifestations with the corresponding time points after myocardial infarction.

(A) < 6 hours
(B) 1 to 3 days
(C) 4 to 6 days
(D) 7 to 14 days

195. Normal gross appearance of myocardium

196. Peak serum levels of myocardial lactate dehydrogenase

197. Beginning of electrocardiographic disturbances

198. Peak tissue infiltration by neutrophils

199. Maximal coagulative necrosis

Questions 200–204

Match each of the following structures with its germ layer of origin.

(A) Ectoderm
(B) Mesoderm
(C) Endoderm
(D) Neuroectoderm

200. Pigment cells of the dermis

201. Adrenal cortex

202. Liver

203. Thyroid gland

204. Gonads

Questions 205–207

Match each description below with the most appropriate abdominal fascia.

(A) Camper's fascia
(B) Scarpa's fascia
(C) Both
(D) Neither

205. Prominent over the abdominal wall

206. Supports sutures

207. Called Colles' fascia in the perineum

Questions 208–212

For each morphologic or functional description of a component of the placenta below, choose the appropriate lettered structure in the accompanying diagram.

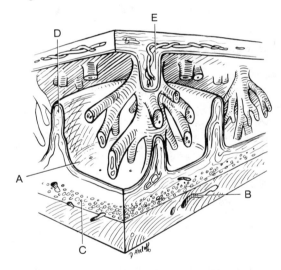

208. This structure is the decidual plate and is penetrated by maternal blood vessels

209. This structure is the intervillous space and contains maternal red blood cells

210. This structure is the chorionic plate and receives the insertion of the umbilical cord

211. This tissue column interconnects the chorionic and decidual plates

212. These structures are chorionic villi and are coated by syncytiotrophoblast

Questions 213–217

Match each procedure or operation with the neurotransmitter that it would deplete.

(A) Serotonin and catecholamines in the cerebral cortex
(B) Gamma-aminobutyric acid (GABA) and glycine in the spinal cord
(C) Substance P in the dorsal horns
(D) Acetylcholine (ACh) in the cerebral cortex
(E) Serotonin in the spinal cord

213. Destruction of spinal interneurons (by controlled hypoxia)

214. Section of dorsal roots

215. Section of the medial forebrain bundle

216. Destruction of the anterior perforated substance

217. Destruction of the medullary raphe

Questions 218–222

Based on the clinical information given below, select the bone tumor that is most likely to occur in each patient.

(A) Osteosarcoma
(B) Chondrosarcoma
(C) Ewing's sarcoma
(D) Giant cell tumor
(E) Osteoid osteoma
(F) Chondroblastoma

218. Epiphyseal lesions in a patient less than 20 years old

219. Epiphyseal lesions in a patient more than 20 years old

220. Metaphyseal lesions in a patient less than 20 years old

221. A radiolucent nidus surrounded by sclerotic bone in a patient less than 20 years old

222. A diaphyseal lesion with concentric onion-skin layering in a patient less than 20 years old

Questions 223–228

Match each disease below with its etiologic agent.

(A) *Treponema pallidum*
(B) *Treponema pertenue*
(C) *Treponema carateum*
(D) *Leptospira interrogans*
(E) *Borrelia recurrentis*

223. Relapsing fever

224. Bejel

225. Pinta

226. Syphilis

227. Fort Bragg fever

228. Yaws

Questions 229–232

Match each visual defect described below with the condition that causes it.

(A) Cataracts
(B) Astigmatism
(C) Presbyopia
(D) Myopia
(E) Hyperopia

229. A progressive decrease in the power of accommodation

230. A progressive loss of lens transparency

231. An optical defect that requires a diverging lens to see distant objects clearly

232. An optical defect that requires continuous accommodation to see distant objects clearly

Questions 233-237

For each function, select the associated transportation protein.

(A) Albumin
(B) Transferrin
(C) Haptoglobin
(D) Transcobalamin
(E) None of the above

233. Iron transport

234. Vitamin B_{12} transport

235. Clot formation

236. Plasma osmotic pressure maintenance

237. Hemoglobin transport

Questions 238-243

The first heart sound (S_1) is composed of sounds from tricuspid and mitral valve closure. The second heart sound (S_2) is the sound of the aortic and pulmonic valves closing. For each cardiovascular abnormality listed below, select the heart sounds with which it is most likely to be associated.

(A) S_1 louder than S_2
(B) S_2 louder than S_1
(C) Aortic valvular ejection sound
(D) Pulmonic valvular ejection sound

238. Mitral valve stenosis

239. Aortic stenosis

240. Acute aortic regurgitation

241. Severe hypertension

242. Anemia

243. Hyperthyroidism

Questions 244-247

For each organ listed below, select the region to which pain in that organ is usually referred.

(A) Inguinal and pubic regions
(B) Perineum, posterior thigh, and leg
(C) Both
(D) Neither

244. Ovary

245. Uterus

246. Epididymis

247. Testis

Questions 248-250

Match each phrase describing a feature of inflammatory heart disease with the disease it characterizes.

(A) Acute rheumatic fever
(B) Chronic rheumatic heart disease
(C) Acute bacterial endocarditis
(D) Subacute bacterial endocarditis
(E) Libman-Sacks endocarditis

248. Fusion of the commissures

249. Infection by group A β-hemolytic streptococci

250. Infection by α-hemolytic (viridans) streptococci

ANSWER KEY

1-B	31-C	61-B	91-C	121-B
2-C	32-B	62-D	92-B	122-C
3-A	33-D	63-E	93-B	123-E
4-C	34-C	64-D	94-C	124-A
5-A	35-C	65-C	95-C	125-B
6-C	36-C	66-E	96-A	126-D
7-A	37-E	67-C	97-B	127-D
8-A	38-E	68-B	98-B	128-D
9-E	39-E	69-E	99-A	129-C
10-E	40-A	70-D	100-B	130-D
11-C	41-D	71-C	101-C	131-C
12-D	42-B	72-B	102-C	132-C
13-C	43-D	73-A	103-B	133-B
14-D	44-B	74-D	104-C	134-A
15-A	45-D	75-C	105-C	135-E
16-C	46-A	76-E	106-C	136-E
17-D	47-C	77-E	107-E	137-A
18-A	48-B	78-D	108-E	138-D
19-B	49-C	79-C	109-A	139-E
20-B	50-B	80-C	110-D	140-B
21-C	51-A	81-D	111-B	141-A
22-A	52-E	82-B	112-E	142-B
23-D	53-D	83-D	113-B	143-D
24-C	54-C	84-B	114-E	144-A
25-C	55-B	85-A	115-C	145-C
26-D	56-A	86-A	116-D	146-B
27-D	57-C	87-D	117-E	147-D
28-D	58-B	88-D	118-B	148-A
29-E	59-A	89-E	119-E	149-C
30-C	60-C	90-A	120-B	150-C

151-B	171-A	191-D	211-B	231-D
152-E	172-D	192-C	212-D	232-E
153-B	173-E	193-A	213-B	233-B
154-C	174-C	194-B	214-C	234-D
155-A	175-B	195-A	215-A	235-E
156-D	176-A	196-B	216-D	236-A
157-C	177-D	197-A	217-E	237-C
158-B	178-C	198-B	218-F	238-A
159-C	179-B	199-B	219-D	239-C
160-D	180-E	200-D	220-A	240-B
161-A	181-E	201-B	221-E	241-B
162-B	182-D	202-C	222-C	242-A
163-D	183-C	203-C	223-E	243-A
164-A	184-B	204-B	224-A	244-A
165-C	185-A	205-C	225-C	245-C
166-E	186-A	206-B	226-A	246-B
167-A	187-C	207-B	227-D	247-A
168-B	188-B	208-C	228-B	248-B
169-D	189-F	209-A	229-C	249-A
170-C	190-E	210-E	230-A	250-D

ANSWERS AND EXPLANATIONS

1. The answer is B. *(Membrane physiology and excitation)* The resting membrane potential is −90 mV, which is primarily due to diffusion potentials caused by K^+ (and Na^+) and the electrogenic Na^+–K^+ pump. Stimulation at time zero [e.g., as occurs with acetylcholine (ACh)] activates a Na^+ channel, thereby greatly increasing Na^+ conductance and leading to depolarization. At the peak of the action potential, the number of open Na^+ channels is 10 times greater than the number of open K^+ channels. Within a short period of time, voltage-gated Na^+ is inactivated, and a K^+ channel opens, greatly increasing the conductance to K^+ and, hence, repolarization. The Ca^{2+}–Na^+ channel (if present) is slow to be activated and normally would depolarize the membrane. Chloride channel permeability does not change during an action potential and, thus, functions passively in this process.

2. The answer is C. *(Gonorrheal and chlamydial coinfections)* Of all cases presenting clinically as gonorrhea, 45% have coexisting chlamydial infections. Therefore, the correct treatment for gonorrhea is the administration of both penicillin for *Neisseria gonorrhoeae* and tetracycline for *Chlamydia trachomatis*. Amoxicillin is an oral penicillin; probenecid increases its blood level by blocking its excretion.

3. The answer is A. *(Immunity to infection)* Opsonic antibodies are important for acquiring immunity to infection by group A *Neisseria meningitidis* because they permit recognition and destruction of *N. meningitidis* at the onset of infection. *Vibrio cholerae*, *Clostridium botulinum*, and *Corynebacterium diphtheriae* exert their pathogenic effects via toxins. Opsonic antibodies are not known to protect against the action of *V. cholerae*, *C. botulinum*, or *C. diphtheriae*.

4. The answer is C. *(Protein metabolism)* Protein kinase C is activated by Ca^{2+} and diacylglycerol (DAG), not by cyclic adenosine monophosphate (cyclic AMP). Cyclic AMP is synthesized from adenosine triphosphate (ATP) in a reaction that is catalyzed by adenylate cyclase. The activity of adenylate cyclase may either be increased or decreased in response to hormone stimulation. Cyclic AMP is the second messenger for the effect of parathyroid hormone (PTH) on the kidney; cyclic AMP also activates protein kinase A. The binding of cyclic AMP to the regulatory subunit results in the dissociation of the regulatory and catalytic subunits and a concomitant increase in protein kinase activity. The degradation of cyclic AMP is mediated by a family of phosphodiesterases, which catalyze the hydrolysis to 5'-AMP.

5 and 6. The answers are: 5-A, 6-C. *(Biostatistical analysis of genetic disorders)* The patient has a brother with poliodystrophy; therefore, the patient's mother and father must be carriers of the disorder. The patient herself may be heterozygous or homozygous for the poliodystrophy gene. The probability that a child born to two known carriers will be healthy is 3/4; the probability that such a child is also a carrier is 1/2. Thus,

$$P \text{ (patient carrier|patient healthy)} = \frac{P \text{ (patient carrier and patient healthy)}}{P \text{ (patient healthy)}}$$
$$= (1/2) \div (3/4)$$
$$= 2/3$$

In the absence of information on his family history of poliodystrophy, the probability that the patient's husband is a carrier is assumed to equal that of the general population (i.e., 1/20). The probability that both the patient and her husband are carriers is, therefore,

$$P \text{ (patient carrier and husband carrier)} = P \text{ (patient carrier)} \, P \text{ (husband carrier)}$$
$$= (2/3)(1/20)$$
$$= 1/30$$

7. The answer is A. *(Pathogenic mechanisms of respiratory pathogens)* Pertussis and diphtheria are caused by *Bordetella pertussis* and *Corynebacterium diphtheriae*, respectively. Both of these pathogens are extracellular bacteria, which adhere to the respiratory tract and produce exotoxins that contribute to pathogenesis. Since *B. pertussis* is gram-negative, it produces endotoxin, unlike gram-positive *C. diphtheriae*. The neurologic problems associated with the DPT vaccine are due to the pertussis component of the vaccine (which uses whole killed cells).

8. The answer is A. *(DNA replication)* DNA replication begins at specific sites. In *Escherichia coli*, DNA replication starts at a unique origin and proceeds sequentially in opposite directions. Multiple replication origins are important for eukaryotic DNA replication. DNA polymerase cannot start chains de novo; all known DNA polymerases add mononucleotides to the 3'-OH end of an RNA primer. Replication requires that the DNA molecule strands must separate and that new daughter strands be synthesized in response to the sequence of bases in the mother strand. This process is called semiconservative replication.

9. The answer is E. *(Diagnosis of pneumonia)* The absence of fever does not exclude infection, especially in very old patients. Physical alterations often precede those on chest film, so the clinician need not invoke a process that changed between examination and radiograph to explain the apparent disparity between the two studies. Tachypnea is not expected with age, and while crackles may be heard in a very few normal individuals at any age, in the context of tachypnea, the clinician must seek another cause.

10. The answer is E. *(Characteristics of volatile anesthetics)* Halothane and methoxyflurane are typical inhalational drugs, which tend to depress both the cardiovascular and respiratory systems. Methoxyflurane is more potent (i.e., it has a lower minimal alveolar concentration) than halothane as predicted from its higher oil:gas partition coefficient (theory of Overton and Meyer). Both result in considerably slower induction than nitrous oxide since their respective blood:gas partition coefficients are greater than that of nitrous oxide. Similarly, recovery from methoxyflurane is slower than that from halothane since its oil:gas partition coefficient is greater than that of halothane. An increase in ventilatory rate will make the onset of anesthesia more rapid for all inhalational anesthetics.

11. The answer is C. *(Acid–base balance)* According to the Henderson-Hasselbalch equation, the patient's pH is approximately 7.4 (normal), and his Pco_2 and $[HCO_3^-]$ are elevated. The elevation in Pco_2 (respiratory acidosis) has been compensated (i.e., normal pH) by a rise in $[HCO_3^-]$. This latter phenomenon is brought about by the kidneys excreting more acid and reabsorbing more HCO_3^-. Full compensation as in this example is most likely to be associated with chronic perturbations in acid–base balance. Such changes may be common in chronic obstructive pulmonary disease (COPD).

12. The answer is D. *(Hassall's corpuscles)* Hassall's (thymic) corpuscles are found in the thymus. They are concentrically laminated structures of unknown function that appear during fetal development and increase in number with age. They are thought to be degenerated medullary epithelial cells and display varying degrees of keratinization or calcification.

13. The answer is C. *(Regulation of arterial blood pressure)* A rise in arterial pressure within the carotid sinus or an increase in pressure secondary to mechanical massage leads to activation of baroreceptors, which subsequently causes inhibition of the central vasoconstrictor center with activation of the central vagal center. The net short-term effect is a decrease in blood pressure, heart rate, and cardiac output. Ultimately, baroreceptors adapt to the stimulus and are unimportant in the long-term regulation of blood pressure. Clamping of the carotid arteries (in a vagotomized animal) will decrease baroreceptor firing and remove inhibitory pathways from the central nervous system (CNS), leading to increases in pressure and heart rate.

14. The answer is D. *(Antioxidants)* Transketolase is a part of the nonoxidative phase of the hexose monophosphate shunt and has no known role in protecting red blood cells from oxygen insult. A number of enzymes are involved in the protection of red blood cells from oxygen insult by H_2O_2 (hydrogen peroxide). Glutathione peroxidase catalyzes the reduction of H_2O_2 to H_2O. The reduced nicotinamide-adenine dinucleotide phosphate (NADPH) utilized by glutathione reductase to regenerate reduced glutathione is produced in the 6-phosphogluconate dehydrogenase reaction. Catalase results in the decomposition of H_2O_2 to water and molecular oxygen.

15. The answer is A. *(Hypocomplementemia-associated renal disease)* Complement levels are normal in immunoglobulin A nephropathy and diffuse proliferative glomerulonephritis (poststreptococcal glomerulonephritis). Nephritides associated with hypocomplementemia include cryoglobulinemia, membranoproliferative glomerulonephropathy, and a variety of visceral infections, including infections of peritoneal and central nervous system (CNS) shunts ("shunt" nephritis).

16. The answer is C. *(Pathogenesis of renal osteodystrophy)* Normally, approximately 90% of serum phosphate is not protein-bound and is, thus, filterable at the glomerulus. Of the filtered phosphate, about 75% is actively reabsorbed, mainly by cotransport with sodium in the proximal tubule. In chronic renal failure, hyperphosphatemia occurs as the glomerular filtration rate (GFR) declines. Hyperphosphatemia produces a secondary hyperparathyroidism as excess phosphate ties up the free serum calcium, in essence leading to hypocalcemia. Vitamin $1,25\text{-}(OH)_2D_3$ levels are reduced directly by the inability of the damaged kidney to convert the $25\text{-}(OH)D_3$, produced by the liver from inactive vitamin D_3, to

1,25-(OH)$_2$D$_3$ and indirectly by the ability of high serum phosphate levels to directly inhibit renal 25-(OH)D$_3$ hydroxylase activity.

17. The answer is D. *(Gram stain; bacterial growth)* Bacterial spores probably caused the decrease in the number of cells expected from the turbidity of the culture. Spores contribute to turbidity, but they do not stain in the Gram procedure.

18. The answer is A. *(Structure and function of amino acids in proteins)* The physical and chemical properties of the peptide reflect the properties of the constituent amino acids. At pH 7.4, the positive and negative charges of the α-amino and α-carboxyl terminal groups cancel one another. The side chains of the two aspartate and one glutamate residues are negatively charged; the side chain of arginine is positively charged. Cysteine and methionine both contain sulfur atoms. Any of the amino acids containing a hydrogen atom attached to a sulfur, nitrogen, or oxygen atom, or containing an atom with an unshared pair of electrons, could form hydrogen bonds. The amino acids valine, phenylalanine, methionine, and cysteine contribute hydrophobic character to the peptide. The specificity of chymotrypsin is for peptide bonds in which the carboxyl group is donated by an aromatic amino acid.

19. The answer is B. *(Energy storage and transfer)* A high-energy bond is defined as a bond that, when hydrolyzed, will release a sufficient amount of energy to drive the synthesis of adenosine triphosphate (ATP) from adenosine diphosphate (ADP) and P$_i$. This requires approximately 7.3 kcal per mole. There are two intermediates in glycolysis that are high-energy compounds: phosphoenolpyruvate and 1,3-bisphosphoglycerate. In the tricarboxylic acid (TCA) cycle, the conversion of succinyl coenzyme A (succinyl CoA) to succinate releases enough energy to synthesize guanosine triphosphate (GTP) from guanosine diphosphate (GDP) and P$_i$. In muscle tissue, phosphocreatine is a storage form of high energy. The hydrolysis of phosphate from phosphocreatine is coupled with the synthesis of ATP. A reaction that is exergonic is accompanied by a $\Delta G°$ that is < 0. The relationship between $\Delta G°$ and K$_{eq}$ is $\Delta G° = -RT \ln K_{eq}$. For a reaction to proceed spontaneously, the K$_{eq}$ must be > 1 and the $\Delta G°$ must be < 0.

20. The answer is B. *(Sodium transport; ATP production)* The ability of erythrocytes to pump Na$^+$ from the cytoplasm depends on a source of adenosine triphosphate (ATP). All of the erythrocyte's ATP is generated by glycolysis. The compound 1,3-diphosphoglycerate is a high-energy glycolytic intermediate which is converted to 3-phosphoglycerate with the concomitant phosphorylation of adenosine diphosphate (ADP) to ATP. This reaction is catalyzed by 3-phosphoglycerate kinase. Pyruvate carboxylase and glucose 6-phosphatase are gluconeogenic enzymes and are not present in the erythrocyte. Malate dehydrogenase is a mitochondrial enzyme and is not present in the erythrocyte. The reaction catalyzed by 6-phosphogluconate dehydrogenase produces reducing power in the reduced form of nicotinamide adenine dinucleotide phosphate (NADPH).

21. The answer is C. *(Toxins; neurotransmission)* The woman is suffering from botulism, which is caused by botulinum neurotoxin. The action of botulinum neurotoxin involves inhibition of acetylcholine (ACh) release from peripheral nerve endings at the neuromuscular junction. Other bacterial toxins have actions described in (A),(B),(D), and (E) [e.g., diphtheria toxin, tetanus toxin, cholera toxin, and streptolysin O, respectively].

22. The answer is A. *(Integral membrane proteins)* Integral membrane proteins are stabilized by hydrophobic interactions between the lipid bilayer and the amino acid side chains. Detergents are required for solubilization. Approximately 20 amino acids in an α-helical conformation are required to span the width of the bilayer. These proteins display compositional asymmetry, with the carbohydrate moieties always being on the side of the membrane away from the cytoplasm. They may display lateral, but not transverse, movement within the membrane.

23. The answer is D. *(Tuberculosis culture; diagnostic tests)* Isolation of *Mycobacterium tuberculosis* is diagnostic of active tuberculosis. The tuberculin test can be positive in the absence of active disease. The clinical findings are not specifically pathognomonic for tuberculosis, nor is demonstration of acid-fast organisms.

24. The answer is C. *(Osteoclasts; bone metabolism)* Osteoclasts are stimulated by parathyroid hormone and inhibited by calcitonin. Osteoclasts are multinucleated cells found on the surface of bone, often in Howship's lacuna. They are bone-resorbing cells involved in remodelling bone and in calcium homeostasis, and probably are derived from the macrophage–monocyte system.

25. The answer is C. *(Regulation of peripheral blood flow)* Compared to other regional vasculatures, the lung is relatively unique in having a vasoconstrictor response to hypoxia rather than a vasodilator response. Although the mechanism remains obscure, the advantage is presumably to improve the matching of ventilation and perfusion by diverting blood flow from poorly ventilated regions of the lung. The heart, like many beds, dilates to adenosine, and this vasodilator mechanism may be common to matching of blood flow to local tissue metabolism. The brain has a very well-described and important vasodilator response to carbon dioxide.

26. The answer is D. *(Therapeutic effects in neoplasia)* Paradoxically, patients with histologically "unfavorable" high-grade lymphomas show long-term survival if a complete clinical remission can be attained. However, it is rare to attain cure in histologically low-grade "favorable" non-Hodgkin's lymphomas: Patients die gradually from bone marrow compromise or lymphoma over many years. Long-term survival after 5 years for diffuse large cell lymphomas is roughly 50%. Those who do not attain complete remission usually die within several years. Spontaneous remissions are rarely seen in aggressive lymphomas.

27. The answer is D. *(Hemoglobin–oxygen interaction)* The affinity of hemoglobin $A_1(\alpha_2\beta_2)$ for oxygen is decreased by an increase in H^+ concentration (a decrease in pH), by an increase in the P_{CO_2}, or by an increase in the concentration of 2,3-diphosphoglycerate (DPG). All of these conditions result in a shift of the oxygen saturation curve to the right. Fetal hemoglobin $(\alpha_2\gamma_2)$ has a higher affinity for oxygen than adult hemoglobin $(\alpha_2\beta_2)$ and consequently becomes saturated at a lower P_{O_2}.

28. The answer is D. *(Chemotherapy and biology of bacteria)* Tetracycline inhibits protein synthesis in bacteria after it is selectively transported inside the cell by an active transport system. Tetracycline is selectively toxic not only because its transport system is peculiar to prokaryotes but also because it binds to 30S subunits of bacterial ribosomes. In bacteria (as well as eukaryote mitochondria), it prevents the binding of charged tRNA to the A site on the ribosomal complex, thereby inhibiting peptide bond synthesis. Thus, it is bacteriostatic, not bactericidal. Resistance can develop secondarily to altered influx or efflux of the drug in prokaryotes. It remains in the gastrointestinal tract and causes its most serious side effects there, either by direct irritation or secondary to modifications in gut flora. This can lead to life-threatening colitis. Tetracycline is hardly ever used in children because it accumulates in developing teeth and bones, causing stains and bone deformities.

29. The answer is E. *(Microcirculation)* Fenestrated capillaries have circular pores (fenestrae), which are 60 nm to 100 nm in diameter and may be partially surrounded by pericytes. The fenestrae often are spanned by a slit diaphragm, which is filamentous and, thus, does not possess a unit membrane structure. Fenestrated capillaries are present in areas where there is a great deal of molecular exchange with blood (e.g., kidney, small intestine, endocrine glands, choroid plexus). Although glomerular capillaries are fenestrated, they lack a slit diaphragm; a thick basement membrane forms the filtration barrier.

30. The answer is C. *(Angina therapy)* Nitroglycerin (glyceryl trinitrate; GTN) is most effective by decreasing preload in angina. At high concentrations, some benefit in angina is obtained from GTN by reducing afterload. However, this latter effect is often accompanied by reflex tachycardia that may disrupt the improvement in myocardial oxygen consumption and supply achieved by GTN. Propranolol is useful in blocking this reflex effect since it is negatively inotropic and negatively chronotropic. Propranolol may be accompanied by coronary artery vasospasm after removing β-receptor–mediated dilation and leaving unopposed a coronary artery α-receptor–mediated vasoconstriction.

31. The answer is C. *(Diagnosis of syphilis)* A Venereal Disease Research Laboratory (VDRL) test and darkfield examination would be the most appropriate combination of tests for determining the cause of the penile lesion. A painless penile lesion that is crateriform, moist, and indurated is suggestive of primary syphilis. The organism responsible, *Treponema pallidum*, cannot be cultured or detected by Gram stain. It can, however, be visualized by darkfield observation of scrapings from the lesion. Some, but not all, patients with primary syphilis have serologic evidence of infection, readily detected by the VDRL test. The fluorescent treponemal antibody absorption (FTA-ABS) test is only used to confirm diagnosis and is not appropriate here.

32–34. The answers are: 32-B, 33-D, 34-C. *(Histology of the epididymis)* The micrograph shows the epididymis. The epididymis is a highly convoluted tubular organ that conveys sperm and fluid from the testis to the ductus (vas) deferens. Its luminal epithelium is a pseudostratified columnar epithelium with numerous tall apical stereocilia. These cells secrete poorly characterized substances, which are added to the seminal fluid, and remove other poorly characterized substances from the fluids that drain from the seminiferous tubules in the testis.

35. The answer is C. *(Inflammation and cellular margination)* As the vascular phase of the inflammatory response progresses, neutrophils and monocytes move toward the periphery of the microcirculatory vessels (a process referred to as margination) and then adhere to, or pavement, the vascular endothelium in preparation for migration into the extravascular space. To migrate, leukocytes develop pseudopods and move, without accompanying loss of fluid, through gaps between the endothelial cells—a process termed diapedesis. In the latter part of the vascular phase, increased vascular permeability causes loss of plasma with resultant venous stasis and, eventually, clotting in the small capillaries local to the inflamed area.

36. The answer is C. *(Zellweger syndrome)* In Zellweger syndrome, the amount of cytosolic catalase is elevated, phytanic acid accumulates in central nervous system (CNS) tissues, the plasma ratio of C26:0/C22:0 fatty acids is elevated, and there is a deficiency of platelet activating factor. Zellweger syndrome results from the absence of or a grossly reduced number of peroxisomes. Peroxisomes are cellular microbodies where oxidation of a very long chain of fatty acids (C26–C40) is initiated, phytanic acid is oxidized, and plasmalogens (such as platelet activating factor) are synthesized.

37. The answer is E. *(Pharmacokinetics of drugs)* Nomograms (i.e., body surface area, creatinine clearance) are reliable indicators of appropriate drug dosages in only about 50% of patients with renal insufficiency. Actual peak and trough levels are the only way to guarantee a therapeutic level of antimicrobial agents and avoid toxicity.

38. The answer is E. *(Gastric carcinoma)* Paget's disease of the breast is a carcinoma involving the nipple and subjacent ductal elements, and Paget's disease of the bone is an idiopathic disease characterized by a high turnover of bone. Neither form is associated with gastric carcinoma. The Leser-Trélat sign is the development of seborrheic keratosis, acanthosis nigricans, or amyloidosis in a patient with gastrointestinal malignancy. Erythema nodosum is seen occasionally with gastrointestinal malignancy.

39. The answer is E. *(Telencephalon)* All of these elements develop from the telencephalon, which includes the internal capsule and the area lateral to it. This area includes the forebrain; parietal, temporal, and occipital lobes; the hippocampus; and the corpus striatum. The thalamus is considered part of the diencephalon.

40. The answer is A. *(Musculature of the oral cavity)* During deglutition, the levator veli palatini muscle raises the soft palate to seal the nasopharynx. Contraction of the palatoglossus elevates the base of the tongue and, with help from the palatopharyngeus muscle, closes the oropharyngeal isthmus behind the food bolus. The superior constrictor muscle helps raise the posterior portion of the pharynx over the bolus.

41. The answer is D. *(Hormone receptors; Addison's disease)* Addison's disease is due to an overall atrophy of the adrenal cortex and is not related to an abnormality in hormone receptors. Many peptide hormone receptors are transmembrane proteins that may elicit their full biologic response when only a small fraction of the receptors are occupied by hormone. The specificity of the response of a particular cell or tissue is defined, at least in part, by the types of receptors localized on or in the cell. Some hormone receptors are desensitized by phosphorylation. Following phosphorylation, dissociation of the hormone from the receptor may occur without a corresponding decrease in the biologic response.

42. The answer is B. *(Asthma; pulmonary mechanics)* The forced vital capacity (FVC) is unchanged or decreased during an acute asthma attack.

43. The answer is D. *(Peptide bonds)* The chemistry of the peptide bond imposes restrictions on higher orders of protein structure. Secondary structure of proteins is stabilized by hydrogen bonds that are formed between the amide hydrogen and carbonyl oxygen of the peptide bond. Because the atoms of the peptide bond lie in a plane, the only rotations that are permissible are around the C_α—C and the N—C_α bonds. There is no formal charge associated with the peptide bond; the electrons of the carbonyl oxygen and the lone pair of electrons on the nitrogen atom are delocalized.

44. The answer is B. *(Mitochondrial intracellular localization)* Mitochondria typically exist in cell areas that use substantial amounts of adenosine triphosphate (ATP). They are abundant in the apices of ciliated cells because the beating action of cilia consumes ATP. They also exist in apices of cells that have a microvillous brush border (e.g., certain kidney cells), because solute transport and pinocytosis of proteins in the glomerular filtrate consume energy and, therefore, require ATP. Mitochondria are distributed evenly throughout the cytoplasm of smooth muscle cells, steroid-secreting cells, skeletal muscle cells, and liver parenchymal cells rather than existing in apical concentrations.

45 and 46. The answers are: 45-D, 46-A. *(Differential diagnosis of infectious mononucleosis)* This patient presents with the classic picture of infectious mononucleosis due to Epstein-Barr virus (EBV) infection. Extreme fatigue, difficulty concentrating, and fever are generalized systemic symptoms. Pharyngitis reflects the local immunologic response by T cells reactive against viral antigens on infected tonsillar B cells. Splenomegaly is also a consequence of immunologic response to EBV. Morphologic examination of lymphocytosis in the peripheral blood should reveal atypical lymphocytes, which are activated T cells with increased cytoplasm and less mature nuclear chromatin. Lymphocytes of infectious lymphocytosis and pertussis are morphologically normal, albeit increased in number; also pertussis is a disease of young children. Serum from this patient should yield a positive test for heterophile antibodies. The combination of pharyngitis and lymphadenopathy are characteristic of EBV-associated mononucleosis. Cytomegalovirus mononucleosis lacks both these features. Toxoplasmosis, a rare cause of mononucleosis, may cause lymphadenopathy but not pharyngitis.

A not uncommon feature of infectious mononucleosis with EBV-mediated expansion of B cells is the development of antibodies to red cells, usually directed against the Ii antigen system. Most such antibodies are cold agglutinins; that is, they react with erythrocytes at temperatures < 37° C. Cold agglutinins are usually of the IgM class, and Coombs' test may or may not be positive. The virus-associated hemophagocytic syndrome has been seen in patients with EBV infections, although usually in immunocompromised patients. Direct infection of erythroid precursors is not a feature of EBV infection. Disseminated intravascular coagulation is a rare occurrence in infectious mononucleosis, and thrombocytopenia may cause petechiae but not hemorrhagic blood loss.

47. The answer is C. *(Glomerular filtration rate)* Blood enters the glomerulus via an afferent arteriole and leaves via an efferent arteriole. A decrease in renal blood flow (RBF) or a decrease in glomerular hydrostatic pressure tends to decrease the glomerular filtration rate (GFR). Accordingly, constriction of the afferent arteriole generally has this effect. An increase in RBF that increases hydrostatic pressure increases GFR. This effect of RBF persists even without an increase in hydrostatic pressure because of a subtle oncotic effect. Although raising systemic pressure would theoretically increase hydrostatic pressure and GFR, the effect is greatly minimized by normal autoregulation in the kidney. Thus, RBF and hydrostatic pressure is maintained by afferent arteriolar constriction in the presence of this increase over normal systemic pressures. Constriction of the efferent arteriole increases hydrostatic pressure (and GFR), but this effect is also offset by the above-mentioned decrease in RBF and, thus, only a modest increase in GFR is normally observed.

48. The answer is B. *(Differential diagnosis of coagulation disorders)* Factor XI deficiency is autosomally transmitted and can result in serious postoperative bleeding, even though it may be mild enough to cause no spontaneous symptoms. Neither factor XII nor Fletcher factor deficiencies result in a bleeding disorder, and inherited factor VIII deficiency occurs only in males. Severe von Willebrand's disease could result in a positive family history and significant bleeding, but rarely is the factor VIII:C low enough to prolong the partial thromboplastin time (PTT), especially when the bleeding time is normal.

49. The answer is C. *(Prokaryotic and eukaryotic differences)* Since shigellas are gram-negative prokaryotic bacteria, they have peptidoglycan-containing cell walls, lipopolysaccharide, 70S ribosomes, RNA, and DNA, but they do not have sterols in their plasma membranes. *Giardia* species are eukaryotic protozoa with 80S ribosomes, RNA, DNA, and sterol-containing plasma membranes.

50–52. The answers are: 50-B, 51-A, 52-E. *(Properties of anesthetic gases)* Minimum alveolar concentration (MAC) is that concentration of anesthetic at 1 atm that produces immobility in 50% of patients exposed to a noxious stimulus.

If an anesthetic has a high blood:gas partition coefficient, it is very soluble in blood and is eliminated from the bloodstream into the alveolar air relatively slowly. This tends to prolong recovery time.

Although there are many plausible theories to explain the action of anesthetic gases, most are based upon the physicochemical properties and the close correlation between the potency of an anesthetic agent and its solubility in oil. There remains no satisfactory explanation as to how these drugs produce general anesthesia.

53. The answer is D. *(Endocrinology)* Growth hormone stimulates cartilage and bone growth via somatomedin, an intermediary peptide. It is secreted periodically, like many other pituitary hormones, and is affected in a negative fashion by somatostatin, a hypothalamic peptide. Unlike other anterior pituitary hormones, cellular targets for growth hormone are relatively ubiquitous. Somatomedin, synthesized in the liver and possibly other sites (e.g., muscle), is an important mediator of the growth effects of the hormone on cartilage and bone. Indeed, growth hormone has no direct effects on these cells by itself. Growth hormone has a large array of effects on amino acid, fat, and carbohydrate activities and, in general, displays anti–insulin-like actions.

54. The answer is C. *(Fluid balance)* Infusion of a hypertonic solution instantaneously adds both volume and milliosmoles to the extracellular (and total body) water space. Because the solution is hypertonic, the osmolality increases in the extracellular space (but remains unchanged in the intracellular space), thereby causing osmosis of water out of the cells and into the extracellular compartment. At equilibrium, the extracellular volume is expanded, and its osmolality is increased. In contrast, the intracellular volume is decreased, resulting in an increase in intracellular osmolality.

55. The answer is B. *(Medical genetics)* Every child has a 50% chance of inheriting a condition with an autosomal dominant mode of inheritance. This does not mean that a family with eight children will necessarily have four affected and four unaffected members, although this is statistically the most likely possibility. It is also possible that all family members will be affected or all will be unaffected, although these possibilities are unlikely.

56. The answer is A. *(Personality assessment)* The major projective instrument of personality assessment is the Rorschach Test. The Thematic Apperception Test, Sentence Completion Test, and projective drawings all are projective tests, but they are less well studied and yield more limited information. The Minnesota Multiphasic Personality Inventory, which is the most frequently used personality test, is an objective instrument, not a projective test.

57. The answer is C. *(Fructosuria; glycogen synthesis)* Essential fructosuria results from a deficiency in fructokinase, which is found only in the liver and catalyzes the first step in the assimilation of fructose by the liver. Under normal conditions, almost all of the fructose is converted to fructose 1-phosphate and is metabolized in the liver. Hexokinase, which is present in all extrahepatic tissues, can convert fructose to fructose 6-phosphate; however, the K_m of hexokinase for fructose is sufficiently high that this reaction does not occur to any significant extent. However, as a consequence of a deficiency in fructokinase, the accumulation of fructose is high enough to be converted to fructose 6-phosphate in extrahepatic tissues and metabolized by the glycolytic pathway. Glucokinase, which is found in the liver, is specific for glucose and cannot catalyze the phosphorylation of fructose. Aldolase B is specific for fructose 1-phosphate. Transketolase is a part of the nonoxidative phase of the pentose phosphate pathway.

58. The answer is B. *(Autonomic pharmacology and effects of antimuscarinic agents)* Atropine may abolish the parasympathetic input that normally maintains a relatively slow heart rate. Indeed, atropine is often used intraoperatively (and in emergencies) to increase heart rate. Atropine inhibits secretions from salivary, lacrimal, bronchial, and sweat glands. It causes mydriasis and cycloplegia. It has no effect on skeletal muscle, in which neuromuscular transmission involves acetylcholine (ACh) and nicotinic, not muscarinic, receptors.

59. The answer is A. *(Presentation of cutaneous erythema)* The etiologic agent of erysipeloid is *Erysipelothrix rhusiopathiae,* a bacterium widely distributed in the environment. Human erysipeloid is clinically described as a slowly spreading cutaneous erythema. Cutaneous edema is characteristic, and the disease is very painful. Cutaneous diphtheria is characterized by a necrotic lesion sometimes associated with insect bites; the bite apparently provides the break in the skin through which toxigenic *Corynebacterium diphtheriae* enters the tissue. Cutaneous nocardiosis is characterized by draining sinus tracts discharging purulent exudate-containing granules. Pontiac fever and listeriosis do not have cutaneous manifestations.

60. The answer is C. *(Knee ligaments)* The medial collateral ligament prevents abduction of the leg at the knee. It extends from the medial femoral epicondyle to the shaft of the tibia. The oblique popliteal ligament resists lateral rotation during the final degrees of extension. The posterior cruciate ligament prevents posterior displacement of the tibia. The anterior cruciate ligament helps lock the knee joint on full extension.

61. The answer is B. *(Nitrogen metabolism)* Negative nitrogen balance would result from defective cholecystokinin-pancreozymin (CCK-PZ) production when the consumption of dietary protein is normal. Negative nitrogen balance occurs when the excretion of nitrogen exceeds the intake of nitrogen. A number of conditions can cause a negative nitrogen balance, including a deficiency in any one of the essential amino acids or a defect in the intestinal phase of protein digestion and absorption. CCK-PZ is essential for stimulating the secretion of inactive pancreatic zymogens, which become active proteases in the small intestine. The intestinal phase of digestion is essential to maintaining nitrogen balance; the gastric phase appears to have little, if any, impact. For example, gastric resection can be performed without affecting nitrogen balance. In phenylketonuria (PKU), tyrosine becomes an essential amino acid and must be supplied in the diet.

62. The answer is D. *(Virulence factors; group A streptococci)* The symptoms and clinical microbiology results indicate that the child has scarlet fever caused by a group A streptococcus *(Streptococcus pyogenes)* infection. This organism causes hemolysis by producing extracellular hemolysins such as streptolysin O. Other important virulence factors of this organism include M protein (which is antiphagocytic and also helps mediate adhesion), lipoteichoic acid (which also mediates adhesion), and a hyaluronic acid capsule. The erythrogenic toxins responsible for scarlet fever rash are not hemolytic.

63. The answer is E. *(Antimicrobials and pseudomembranous colitis)* The patient is likely suffering from antibiotic-associated pseudomembranous colitis (note the patient's diarrhea and deterioration following antibiotic therapy). Sigmoidoscopic examination, Gram stain of feces for white blood cells, ordering a *Clostridium difficile* toxin test, and isolating the patient are appropriate procedures to follow for a patient suspected of having antibiotic-associated pseudomembranous colitis caused by *C. difficile*. However, changing the antibiotic from a cephalosporin to clindamycin is inappropriate because *C. difficile* is not sensitive to clindamycin.

64. The answer is D. *(Enteric infection by enterotoxigenic bacteria)* The symptoms of cholera result from the attachment of *Vibrio cholerae* to the intestinal mucosa and production of cholera toxin. The infection is acute, and the bacteria remain extracellular. The action of cholera toxin involves elevation of intestinal cyclic AMP levels, which results in massive fluid loss (seen as diarrhea).

65. The answer is C. *(Sterilization; disinfection)* Bacterial endospores are the life forms most resistant to heat, and they can survive boiling for several minutes. Medically important endospore-formers include members of the genera *Bacillus* and *Clostridium*.
 Non–spore-formers such as *Escherichia coli* and *Mycobacterium tuberculosis* are more heat-sensitive than spore-formers and are usually killed after several minutes of boiling.

66. The answer is E. *(Cushing's syndrome)* Cushing's syndrome may be caused by hypothalamic or pituitary pathology or both, adrenal adenoma (or carcinoma), and exogenous glucocorticoid administration. Hypersecretion of adrenocorticotropic hormone (ACTH) from the pituitary gland, due to either an underlying tumor or overstimulation from corticotropin releasing factor (CRF) of hypothalamic origin, will stimulate a responsive adrenal cortex to release excess amounts of glucocorticoids (and mineralocorticoids). Other sites of excessive ACTH secretion, including tumors of nonendocrine origin, may be important. A useful initial screen to detect the presence of the syndrome is to inject dexamethasone and then to monitor the expected suppression of cortisol (due to pituitary inhibition) in plasma the following day. Patients with various forms of Cushing's syndrome and a responsive adrenal cortex will not undergo the predicted suppression until considerably higher amounts of dexamethasone are administered. Subsequent tests [including urinary secretion and administration of metyrapone (cortisol synthesis inhibitor)] and diagnostic procedures will help identify the source of the excessive cortisol production.

67–73. The answers are: 67-D, 68-B, 69-E, 70-D, 71-C, 72-B, 73-A. *(Skeletal muscular anatomy and properties of halothane)* Unlike intravenous anesthetics (e.g., methohexital), inhalational anesthetics such as halothane do not possess notable excitatory effects on the central nervous system (CNS). All anesthetics tend to depress cardiac function and respiratory drive. Halothane and other anesthetics may induce malignant hyperthermia in certain genetically susceptible individuals.
 The anterior cruciate ligament (ACL) is important to the proper functioning of the knee joint. The ACL attaches the femur to the tibia. Damage to this ligament is usually sports-related and due to rapid deceleration or torque. The ligament is essential to the stability of the knee joint, and surgery is necessary to prevent further injury.
 Latin for "little vinegar saucer," the acetabulum is the rounded cavity on the external surface of the innominate bone that receives the head of the femur.

The epiphyseal plate lies between the epiphysis and diaphysis of long bones and is the area of highest mitotic activity. During bone growth, the epiphyseal plates migrate distally, finally becoming epiphyseal lines when growth is completed.

The cuboid is a tarsal bone. The navicular is both a carpal and a tarsal bone. All of the other bones listed (i.e., capitate, trapezium, trapezoid) are carpal bones.

A haversian system, or osteon, is made up of osteocytes, lacunae, canaliculi, and concentric lamellae. It is the fundamental unit of compact bone.

74. The answer is D. *(Enzyme inhibition)* The data in the Lineweaver-Burk plot are diagnostic of noncompetitive inhibition. The intercept on the 1/[S] axis indicates that the inhibitor has no effect on the K_m for the substrate. The increase in the 1/v intercept observed in the presence of the inhibitor indicates a decrease in the V_{max} of the reaction. Noncompetitive inhibitors interact at a site other than the active site. They usually bear no structural resemblance to either the substrate or the transition-state analogs, and their effects cannot be reversed by high concentrations of substrates. Competitive inhibitors, however, interact at the active site, are structurally related to transition-state analogs, and can be reversed by high concentrations of substrate.

75. The answer is C. *(Urea metabolism; amino acid enzymes)* The pathway by which the α-amino groups of the amino acids are incorporated into urea involves a number of transaminases that transfer the amino group from the amino acids to α-ketoglutarate, with the concomitant formation of glutamate. The glutamate is converted back to α-ketoglutarate and NH_4^+ by the mitochondrial enzyme glutamate dehydrogenase. The NH_4^+ produced in the reaction is the substrate for carbamoyl phosphate synthesis. This reaction constitutes the first step in urea biosynthesis.

76. The answer is E. *(Allosteric enzymes)* Allosteric enzymes have sites distinct from the active site where regulatory ligands bind and alter either the V_{max} or the K_m for the substrate. The substrate saturation curves do not obey Michaelis-Menten kinetics and frequently show sigmoidicity, which is indicative of positive cooperativity between active sites. Enzymes that obey Michaelis-Menten kinetics require an 81-fold increase in substrate concentration to achieve an increase from 10% to 90% of the V_{max}. Allosteric enzymes that display positive cooperativity require a smaller increase in substrate concentration to achieve the same increase in V_{max}. The allosteric sites may be located either on the same subunit as the catalytic site or on a separate regulatory subunit. Enzymes with these regulatory properties frequently catalyze reactions that are either rate-limiting or occupy a pivotal point in a metabolic pathway.

77. The answer is E. *(Chronic obstructive pulmonary disease)* Risk for chronic obstructive pulmonary disease (COPD) with various degrees of emphysema or chronic bronchitis is strongly associated with cigarette smoking and exposure to irritating substances in the environment (e.g., sulfur dioxide) or workplace (e.g., silica, cotton or grain dust, toluene diisocyanate). Usually, it is associated with older age-groups, especially individuals with preexisting lung disease. A genetically linked deficiency in α_1-antitrypsin is strongly linked to premature obstructive pulmonary disease. Although intravenous drug abuse is associated with pulmonary complications, including acute respiratory failure and opportunistic infections accompanying immunodeficiency-like syndromes in certain individuals, it is not usually considered a risk factor for COPD.

78. The answer is D. *(Angiotensin-converting enzyme inhibitors)* Captopril is the prototype of a group of angiotensin-converting enzyme (ACE) inhibitors. These agents lower blood pressure in poorly understood ways, but a critical role for inhibition of ACE (with loss of production of angiotensin II) seems apparent. ACE inhibitors do not affect renin per se, nor do they have any activity towards angiotensin II receptors.

79. The answer is C. *(Neoplasia and hormone action)* Tamoxifen has become the drug of choice for the initial endocrine management of breast cancer as well as a useful adjuvant therapy for the palliative management of advanced breast cancer. It is relatively nontoxic, and patients with breast tumors containing estrogen receptors are most likely to respond to the drug. The drug binds to the estrogen receptor in the nucleus but does not stimulate transcription. The tamoxifen–estrogen receptor complex does not readily dissociate, thereby affecting estrogen receptor recycling. In premenopausal women, competition with estrogen receptors in the anterior pituitary and hypothalamus disrupts normal feedback inhibition of gonadotropin-releasing hormone, thereby enhancing gonadotropin release.

80. The answer is C. *(Neuromuscular transmission)* Motoneurons innervate many skeletal muscle fibers. In large muscles, thousands of fibers may be innervated by one neuron. However, each fiber receives only one axon terminal. Depolarization of the nerve terminal releases acetylcholine (ACh) into the synaptic cleft, where it binds directly to Na$^+$ channels, causing an end-plate potential. The end-plate itself is not electrically excitable, but passive spreading of end-plate potential to a nearby membrane leads to propagation of the action potential and contraction of all muscle fibers innervated by the motoneuron. When ACh is the neurotransmitter, termination of transmission is accomplished by hydrolysis via acetylcholinesterase.

81–82. The answers are: 81-D, 82-B. *(Volume of distribution; pharmacokinetics; half-life of elimination)* The volume of distribution (V_d) is approximately 10 L. V_d is defined as

$$V_d = \text{dose}/Cp$$

where Cp is the plasma concentration at zero time. In this case, the Cp can be estimated easily because the log plasma concentration versus time plot is linear; it is approximately 100 μg/ml. Thus,

$$V_d = \frac{(20 \text{ mg/kg}) (50 \text{ kg})}{0.1 \text{ mg/ml}}$$
$$= 10,000 \cdot \text{ml}$$
$$= 10 \text{ L}$$

The half-life of elimination of this drug was approximately 4 hours. The half-life of elimination can be determined graphically from the slope of the linear plot. First, note the time when a given concentration (e.g., 50 μg/ml) was detected (5 hours). Next, determine the time when half the original value (25 μg/ml) was detected (9 hours). Then, calculate the half-life of elimination: $9 - 5 = 4$ hours.

83. The answer is D. *(Structure and function of proteins)* The chemical properties of proteins are determined by the nature of the constituent amino acid side chains. Only L-amino acids are incorporated into proteins. The participation of the amide nitrogen of proline in a cyclic ring structure prohibits the formation of hydrogen bonds, and disrupts α-helical structure. There are no ionizing groups on the side chain of glutamine to provide buffering capacity; the isoelectric pH (pI) of both aspartate and glutamate is approximately 4.5.

84. The answer is B. *(Pathophysiology of idiopathic thrombocytopenic purpura)* Idiopathic thrombocytopenic purpura (ITP) is most common in young women, and the usual presentation is of isolated thrombocytopenia without associated illness. Amegakaryocytic thrombocytopenia can occur, but it is much less common, especially in this age-group. Drug-induced thrombocytopenia is also possible but is unlikely in a healthy woman who has no reason to take medications. Patients with thrombasthenia are not thrombocytopenic, and aleukemic leukemia is unlikely to occur without other cytopenias.

85. The answer is A. *(Pathophysiology of anemia)* Diets deficient in vitamin B_{12} or folate can result in macrocytic, normochromic anemia with characteristic hypersegmented neutrophils. Anemia due to folate or vitamin B_{12} deficiency often also presents with thrombocytopenia and agranulocytopenia. Microcytic, hypochromic erythrocytes are observed in iron deficiency anemia and thalassemia minor. Additionally, basophilic stippling and target cells can be seen in thalassemia minor. In sickle cell crisis, the anemia is normocytic and normochromic, as is the anemia associated with hemorrhage.

86. The answer is A. *(RNA structure and function)* The synthesis of RNA in eukaryotes requires three different RNA polymerases; one each for the synthesis of mRNA, rRNA, and tRNA. All of these RNAs are required for protein synthesis. The ribosome is a complex made up of approximately 75 proteins and several types of rRNA and is the site where mRNA and tRNAs come together to participate in protein synthesis. The triplet base codons for amino acids are contained in mRNA; tRNA contains a complementary anticodon, which promotes interaction between mRNA and tRNA during protein synthesis.

87. The answer is D. *(Respiratory epithelium)* Clara cells are primarily found in the terminal and respiratory bronchioles and may help metabolize inhaled toxins. The trachea, extrapulmonary bronchi, and intrapulmonary bronchi are primarily composed of ciliated, mucous, enteroendocrine, and basal cells. Alveoli are composed of type I and type II pneumocytes.

88. The answer is D. *(RNA structure and function)* The primary transcript for mRNAs is formed in the nucleus, where the elongation proceeds from the 5' to the 3' end. Most eukaryotic mRNAs are distinctive in that the 5' ends are capped by the addition of a methylated guanylic acid residue and the 3' ends have a polyadenylate tail of 100 to 200 adenosine nucleotides. Most precursor forms of mRNA contain intervening sequences, which are removed by a process known as splicing. The binding of steroid hormones with their receptors to specific genes results in the increased synthesis of the mRNA encoded in those genes.

89. The answer is E. *(Gluconeogenesis and glycolysis)* Stimulation of beta cells by glucose results in the release of insulin. Insulin has numerous effects on virtually every tissue, and its overall effect is the conservation of body fuel supplies. It does this by promoting the uptake and storage of glucose, amino acids, and fats. In the liver, it decreases gluconeogenesis and glycogenolysis and promotes glycolysis. In addition, it promotes lipogenesis in the liver and fat and is antilipolytic. It is also an important anabolic protein hormone while simultaneously inhibiting the breakdown of amino acids. It inhibits the release of glucagon from neighboring alpha cells.

90. The answer is A. *(Glycolysis)* The primary site of glycolysis regulation is the conversion of fructose 6-phosphate to fructose 1,6-bisphosphate. The enzyme, 1-phosphofructokinase, is an allosteric enzyme that is inhibited by adenosine triphosphate (ATP) and citrate and is activated by fructose 2,6-bisphosphate. The concentration of fructose 2,6-bisphosphate is, in turn, regulated by glucagon. Acetylcoenzyme A (CoA) is not an allosteric effector of any of the glycolytic enzymes. Glucose 6-phosphate is an inhibitor of hexokinase.

91. The answer is C. *(Pharmacologic treatment of arrhythmias)* Lidocaine is often the drug of first choice for the treatment of ventricular arrhythmia since it has a predilection to suppress Na^+ channels of cardiac cells in the infarct area that have abnormal resting membrane potentials and elevated K^+ levels. In addition, lidocaine is more selective for the faster, more activated channels, as in the case of ventricular tachycardia, than for the normally slower conducting Na^+ channels. If lidocaine fails, the most frequently chosen agent is another Na^+-channel blocker, procainamide. The Ca^{2+}-channel blockers (diltiazem, verapamil) and β-blockers (propranolol) have a greater effect on supraventricular disturbances where slow Ca^{2+} channels are more significantly involved.

92. The answer is B. *(Mechanics of the heart)* At the end of the period of isovolumic contraction (2), the pressure inside the ventricle has risen to equal the pressure in the aorta at end diastole (80 mm Hg). At this point, ventricular pressures push the aortic valve open, and blood begins to pour out of the left ventricle (3) while it continues to contract. The fraction of end diastolic volume (115 ml) that was ejected was 60% since stroke volume was 115 − 45 = 70 ml. After isovolumic relaxation, left ventricular end diastolic pressure was near atmospheric pressure.

93. The answer is B. *(Innervation of the genitourinary and gastrointestinal tracts)* Afferents from the kidneys, upper ureters, and gonads travel through the aorticorenal plexus along the upper lumbar splanchnic nerves. The uterus, midureter, and descending and sigmoid colons send nerve fibers to the aortic plexus along the lumbar splanchnic nerves. Pain from these structures is referred to the inguinal region. Visceral afferent nerves from the bladder, cervix, lower ureters, rectum, and superior anal canal traverse the pelvic splanchnic nerves and travel through the pelvic plexus to the spinal cord. Pain is referred along the dermatomes S2–S4 to the leg, foot, and perineum.

94. The answer is C. *(Antiphagocytic virulence factors)* Opsonizing antibodies promote phagocytosis and are often directed against the capsules of pathogens, including *Streptococcus pneumoniae*. The most important function of the *S. pneumoniae* capsule is to inhibit phagocytosis (until opsonizing antibodies are produced). The capsules of both *Hemophilus influenzae* type B and *Neisseria meningitidis* are polysaccharides that elicit a poor T-cell–dependent immune response. The existing DPT vaccine contains killed whole *Bordetella pertussis* cells, not purified capsules.

95. The answer is C. *(Gastrointestinal transport of fats)* The formation of fatty acids and monoglyceride by pancreatic lipase is an important step in the digestive fate of triglycerides. Although there are gastric lipases, they have a relatively insignificant effect on ingested neutral fats. This is in contrast to a critical role for pancreatic lipase in the pancreatic juice. Neutral fats are emulsified by bile salts, and further agitation within the intestine makes their surface available for significant hydrolysis by the water-soluble pancreatic lipase. The products, fatty acids and 2-monoglyceride, would quickly convert back to fat if they were not made into micelles by bile salts. These bile salts ferry the micelles to the intestinal brush border where the hydrophobic fatty acid (and monoglyceride) rapidly diffuse passively through the lipid membrane.

96. The answer is A. *(Autonomic pharmacology)* Indirect-acting sympathomimetic agents, like amphetamine, are transported into nerve terminals by the uptake 1 mechanism where they displace norepinephrine to account for the pressor response. Because these agents lack hydroxyl groups on the catechol ring, they are without significant direct effects on synaptic receptors. Thus, their action is affected by the presence of other agents that modify adrenergic transmission. Reserpine depletes norepinephrine stores, and monoamine oxidase (MAO) inhibitors may potentiate norepinephrine levels. Thus, the pressor response to amphetamine would be potentiated by an MAO inhibitor and decreased by reserpine. Imipramine interferes with uptake of amphetamine and reduces its effect in this and other ways. A hallmark of indirect-acting sympathomimetics is tolerance or tachyphylaxis. This is presumably secondary to depletion of endogenous norepinephrine pools after repetitive application of amphetamine.

97. The answer is B. *(Urea cycle)* The nitrogens in urea, the disposal form of ammonia, come from ammonia and aspartate. Ammonia reacts with carbon dioxide and adenosine triphosphate (ATP) to form carbamoyl phosphate in a reaction catalyzed by carbamoyl phosphate synthetase (ammonia). This enzyme requires N-acetylglutamate as a positive allosteric effector. Without this reaction, urea would not be formed, and ammonia levels would be high. The next step in the urea cycle is the reaction of carbamoyl phosphate with ornithine to form citrulline. In the absence of carbamoyl phosphate, ornithine levels are high, citrulline is undetectable, and neither argininosuccinate nor arginine is formed.

98. The answer is B. *(Oxidative enzymes)* The extraction of β-hydroxybutyrate from blood, and its oxidation to CO_2 and H_2O, requires the participation of acetoacetate thiokinase and β-hydroxybutyrate dehydrogenase. All tissues except the liver use β-hydroxybutyrate as a metabolic fuel. The three enzymes required for catabolism of the ketone bodies are localized in the mitochondria. These enzymes are: β-hydroxybutyrate dehydrogenase; succinyl CoA: acetoacetate acyltransferase; and acetoacetate thiokinase. Hydroxymethylglutaryl coenzyme A (HMG CoA) lyase catalyzes a step in fatty acid oxidation that takes place in the kidneys or liver. HMG CoA lyase breaks down *(S)*-3-hydroxy-3-methyl-glutaryl-CoA into acetyl CoA and acetoacetate.

99. The answer is A. *(Neutropenia and infection)* Neutropenia is defined as an absolute neutrophil count $< 1500/\mu l$. While there is a modest risk of acquired infection beginning at this level, patients with neutrophil counts of $< 1000/\mu l$ for any length of time are at significant risk of acquired infection and patients below $500/\mu l$ are at extreme risk. The peripheral blood differential count percentages are of limited value. They must be multiplied times the total white cell count to arrive at absolute numbers of circulating granulocytes, monocytes, and lymphocytes. Leukocyte percentages determined by a 100-cell manual differential count have extremely broad 95% confidence intervals that may yield broad apparent shifts in absolute numbers. New cell counters with machine analysis of % neutrophils, monocytes, and lymphocytes (even eosinophils and basophils) offer a better estimate of absolute number.

100. The answer is B. *(DNA and restriction enzymes)* Restriction enzymes recognize specific base sequences in double-helical DNA and cleave both strands of the duplex at specific sites. Most of the cleavage sites contain a twofold rotational symmetry (the recognized sequence is palindromic). The cuts resulting from these enzymes may be either staggered or blunt. Restriction enzymes can cleave DNA molecules into a number of specific fragments. These enzymes are specific for DNA; they do not cleave RNA.

101. The answer is C. *(Human genetics and Duchenne muscular dystrophy)* In Duchenne muscular dystrophy (DMD) the amount of dystrophin (a 400 kD protein of unknown function, but thought to be involved in calcium regulation) is reduced from its normal 0.002% of total protein. Derangement of calcium homeostasis is thought to be the cause of the excessive shortening of the sarcomeres. The affected muscle groups hypertrophy due to replacement of muscle mass by fibrofatty tissue. DMD is most often transmitted from a female carrier to the affected male (about 1 per 3500 live-born males) by X-linked recessive inheritance (myotonic dystrophy is associated with mutations on chromosome 19), although approximately one-third of the cases appear to be due to spontaneously arising mutations.

102. The answer is C. *(Pathophysiology of anthrax)* A malignant pustule is a clinical manifestation of cutaneous anthrax. It occurs at the site of inoculation and is characterized by a black eschar at its base surrounded by an inflamed ring. Enteritis necroticans caused by *Clostridium perfringens* and pseudomembranous colitis caused by *Clostridium difficile* are diseases of the gastrointestinal tract that may be characterized by ulcerative lesions in the intestinal mucosa. Lockjaw is a lay name for tetanus; it refers to the muscle and neural spasms caused by the neurotoxin tetanospasmin. Woolsorter's disease is pulmonary anthrax—a diffuse, lethal, progressive pneumonia caused by the inhalation of spores of *Bacillus anthracis*.

103. The answer is B. *(Amino acid catabolism)* The amount of alanine released from skeletal muscle is greater than the amount that can be accounted for in muscle protein. The catabolism of many amino acids in muscle involves the transamination of α-amino groups from amino acids to pyruvate as an acceptor. The product of this reaction is alanine. Thus, the carbon skeleton of much of the alanine released from muscle is derived from glucose via the glycolytic pathway.

104. The answer is C. *(Antibiotic action)* Chloramphenicol is bacteriostatic, and, therefore, was responsible for the leveling off of curve A. All of the agents listed, except chloramphenicol, are bactericidal. Cephalothin, methicillin, and vancomycin all interfere with cell wall synthesis, leading to bursting and to cell death. Polymyxin affects cell membrane function, causing irreversible loss of small molecules from the cell. Chloramphenicol inhibits protein synthesis and is bacteriostatic. Hence, the cell number in the culture with chloramphenicol does not decrease, and the organisms are viable. Removal of chloramphenicol will result in growth.

105. The answer is C. *(Membrane structure and function)* The plasma membrane consists of amphipathic lipids (predominately phospholipids and cholesterol) and amphipathic proteins. The hydrophilic portions of these molecules face the external and internal aqueous environments. The hydrophobic portions are in the internal portion of the bilayer. Phospholipids prevent free diffusion of ions and water-soluble molecules, thereby imparting selective permeability properties to the lipid bilayer. Proteins may be restricted to the external portion of the bilayer or span its entirety. In addition, the membrane is fluid, allowing lateral diffusion of even large proteins.

106–107. The answers are: 106-C, 107-E. *(Bacterial meningitis)* The findings of fever, headache, nuchal rigidity, and lethargy with an acute onset and the lack of dramatic neurologic manifestations suggest acute bacterial meningitis. Viral meningitis causes much of the same symptomatology, but the onset typically is more insidious and the patient usually is less acutely ill. Patients with viral encephalitis display the same general symptomatology as those with viral meningitis, but encephalitis is differentiated by dramatic neurologic manifestations and a much poorer prognosis. Fungal meningitis is more chronic and frequently is seen with other systemic signs of mycotic disease. Brain abscess usually is seen with other foci of infection, and the patient typically has deficits that reflect the location of the lesion.

Streptococcus pneumoniae is the most common cause of bacterial meningitis among the elderly. *Hemophilus influenzae* type b is the most common cause of bacterial meningitis overall. Its incidence is highest in children 6 to 12 months old and decreases with age; the incidence of meningitis caused by *H. influenzae* is low in adults. Meningococcal meningitis occurs primarily among young adults, and *Neisseria meningitidis* serogroups A, B, C, and Y cause most cases. *Staphylococcus aureus* occasionally causes meningitis but is a common cause of brain abscess.

108. The answer is E. *(Cholesterol biosynthesis)* The synthesis of cholesterol utilizes acetyl CoA as the sole source of carbon atoms and reduced nicotinamide-adenine dinucleotide phosphate (NADPH) as a source of reducing equivalents. The NADPH is supplied primarily through two reactions, which are catalyzed by a glucose 6-phosphate dehydrogenase and 6-phosphogluconate dehydrogenase. The formation of HMG CoA results from the condensation of acetoacetyl CoA and acetyl CoA. The step that is committed to cholesterol synthesis is the conversion of HMG CoA to mevalonic acid. This step is catalyzed by HMG CoA reductase. HMG CoA is used to synthesize activated isoprenoid units, which are subsequently condensed to form squalene. Squalene is converted to lanosterol and then to cholesterol by a series of reactions that involve the addition of oxygen, cyclization to give the sterol ring structure, and elimination of three carbon atoms as CO_2. Mevinolin is an inhibitor of HMG CoA reductase.

109. The answer is A. *(Skeletal muscle)* The length of the A band remains constant during the contraction of myofibrils in skeletal muscle. The sarcomere of the myofibril is composed of thick and thin filaments. According to the sliding filament hypothesis, thick and thin filaments slide past one another during contraction, increasing the amount of overlap between them; they do not change length. The H band contains only thick filaments; the A band contains thin and thick filaments. The I band contains only thin filaments, which are anchored in the middle of the I band by components of the Z disk. During contraction, thin filaments slide into the A band, reducing the size of both the H band and I band and drawing the Z disks closer to the A band.

110. The answer is D. *(Renal sodium transport)* Almost 75% of Na^+ is reabsorbed in the proximal tubular epithelium by several processes, including: active transport at the basolateral surface leading to electrogenic potential with additional passive movement; and cotransport of Na^+ at the luminal surface with glucose or amino acids. An additional 22% is reabsorbed by the active transport process in the ascending thick limb of the loop of Henle. The remaining small percent of Na$^+$ that reaches the distal tubular epithelium is reabsorbed by a highly regulated aldosterone-sensitive process involving exchange with K$^+$.

111. The answer is B. *(Tumor pathology)* In most human cancers, the stage of the disease is the most important prognostic factor. Stage refers to the extent, or degree of spread, of the disease in the patient (i.e., localized, regional, or distant). Tumor grade (i.e., differentiation), mitotic count, and extent of invasion correlate with the stage of the tumor, in that higher-grade (i.e., less differentiated) tumors and highly invasive tumors tend to be higher-stage lesions.

112. The answer is E. *(Microbiology)* The principles of antibiotic action are perhaps best exemplified by penicillin. Antibiotics often act by specifically binding to macromolecules only found in the parasite. Transpeptidase is the only penicillin-binding protein listed; it is inactivated when binding occurs.

113. The answer is B. *(Enteric infections)* **Salmonella typhi** is a highly invasive pathogen that is readily disseminated throughout the body. In typhoid fever, this organism invades through the intestinal mucosa and spreads through the body via the lymphatic system. In nontyphoid *Salmonella* infections, the bacteria invade into the intestinal submucosa but usually do not spread into other regions of the body. *Campylobacter jejuni* and *Shigella dysenteriae* invade the intestinal mucosa but usually do not penetrate the submucosa or spread throughout the body. *Vibrio cholerae* is noninvasive.

114. The answer is E. *(Gram-negative pathogens; intracellular pathogens)* **Salmonella typhi** is an intracellular pathogen; therefore, gentamicin is ineffective against the enteric fevers caused by the organisms. *Hemophilus influenzae* type B epiglottitis, *Pseudomonas aeruginosa* burn infections, *Klebsiella pneumoniae* respiratory infections, and *Escherichia coli* urinary tract infections are caused by extracellular pathogens.

115. The answer is C. *(Gluconeogenesis)* Gluconeogenesis utilizes the enzymes in glycolysis that catalyze reversible reactions. The enzymes that catalyze irreversible steps in glycolysis are hexokinase, 1-phosphofructokinase, and pyruvate kinase. In order to circumvent the three irreversible reactions, the de novo synthesis of glucose requires four enzymes that are unique to gluconeogenesis: pyruvate carboxylase, phosphoenolpyruvate carboxykinase (PEPCK), fructose 2,6-bisphosphatase, and glucose 6-phosphatase.

116. The answer is D. *(Properties of tricyclic antidepressants)* Tricyclic antidepressants, such as imipramine, inhibit neuronal uptake of norepinephrine, serotonin, and other central nervous system (CNS) amines. Potentiation of local concentrations of these amines may underlie the ability of these agents to reverse symptoms of depression after chronic administration over several weeks. The parent and metabolite compounds of many of these drugs can directly or indirectly affect cardiac function (including α-adrenergic receptor blockade) and, thus, may cause orthostatic hypotension and cardiac dysrhythmias. Indeed, suicide with these agents is quite common, and the cause of death is related to cardiac toxicity. The drugs do not appear to affect dopamine receptors significantly in the concentrations used clinically. Some agents are more selective for serotonin uptake (fluoxetine) than for norepinephrine uptake (desipramine).

117. The answer is E. *(RNA structure and function)* In eukaryotes, the mRNA is formed in the nucleus and must be exported into the cytosol for translation. The initial product of transcription includes all of the introns and flanking regions, which must be removed by splicing before correct translation can occur. The splicing reaction involves hydrolysis of phosphodiester bonds and formation of new phosphodiester bonds within the mRNA molecule. Other processing reactions include additions at both the 5' and 3' ends. A guanosine triphosphate (GTP) molecule is added in reverse orientation to form a cap at the 5' end, and the cap is further modified by the addition of methyl groups. At the 3' end a polyadenylate tail is added.

118. The answer is B. *(Protein synthesis)* Protein synthesis occurs in both the cytoplasm and the mitochondria of cells and requires large amounts of energy. In addition to requiring ATP for the formation of aminoacyl tRNA, guanosine triphosphate (GTP) is required for initiation, formation, translocation, and termination of the peptide bond. Protein synthesis requires mRNA, tRNA, and rRNA. Peptide-bond formation involves the transfer of the nascent polypeptide chain from one tRNA to the amino group of another aminoacyl tRNA. This reaction is accomplished by the enzyme complex known as peptidyltransferase, which is an integral part of the 50S ribosomal subunits.

119. The answer is E. *(Protein synthesis)* The synthetic polynucleotide sequence of CAACAACAACAA... could be read by the in vitro protein synthesizing system starting at the first C, the first A, or the second A. In the first case, the first triplet codon would be CAA, which codes for glutamine. In the second case, the first triplet would be AAC, which codes for asparagine; and in the last case, the triplet would be ACA, which would have to be a codon for threonine.

120. The answer is B. *(Mycology) Cryptococcus neoformans* is responsible for meningitis in this case. The india ink microscopic staining technique demonstrated the presence of yeast cells producing a capsule (the capsule appears as a clear halo), and the only encapsulated yeast among the options is *C. neoformans*. This organism is an important fungal cause of meningitis, and it often infects AIDS patients.

121. The answer is B. *(Mycobacteria) Mycobacterium tuberculosis* produces factors such as sulfatides, which inhibit the fusion of phagosomes with lysosomes. In addition to inhibition of phagosome–lysosome fusion, *M. tuberculosis* escapes cell killing by lysosomal factors. The organisms are also resistant to phagocytic killing due to their tough cell surface.

122–129. The answers are: 122-C, 123-E, 124-A, 125-B, 126-D, 127-D, 128-D, 129-C. *(Neuromuscular transmission and pathophysiology and treatment of myasthenia gravis)* Edrophonium is a short-acting acetylcholinesterase inhibitor, which increases synaptic acetylcholine (ACh) levels. An increase in muscle strength upon administration of edrophonium is diagnostic of myasthenia gravis.

Myasthenia gravis is a neuromuscular disorder with muscle weakness due to blockade of ACh receptors by autoantibodies to the ACh receptors. The antibody–receptor complex is incapable of responding to ACh and is also rapidly internalized and degraded.

Although the mechanism of action is unclear, aminoglycoside antibiotics and Ca^{2+} have opposing actions in a variety of organ systems. Thus, Ca^{2+} attenuates both the ototoxicity and nephrotoxicity of the aminoglycosides, and the aminoglycosides inhibit presynaptic release of ACh, a process known to be Ca^{2+}-dependent. Intravenous administration of a calcium salt is the preferred treatment for aminoglycoside-induced neuromuscular blockade. Citrate, an anticoagulant, chelates divalent metals and would, therefore, not be useful.

Penicillamine is an effective chelator of heavy metals and is used for the treatment of copper, lead, and mercury poisoning. One of the unusual long-term side effects of penicillamine is a muscle weakness that is indistinguishable from myasthenia gravis.

About 65% of patients with myasthenia gravis have a hyperplastic thymus, and another 10% have a thymic tumor (thymoma). Surgical removal of the thymus and tumors often improves the symptoms dramatically.

Pyridostigmine is the medium-term acetylcholinesterase inhibitor most commonly used to treat myasthenia gravis. Isoflurophate (di*iso*propyl phosphorofluoridate; DFP) is an irreversible acetylcholinesterase inhibitor whose use is limited to ophthalmic applications; pralidoxime is the rationally designed cholinesterase reactivator that is antidotal for organophosphorus poisoning; and triorthocresylphosphate, the adulterant in Jamaican ginger, was the organophosphorus poison responsible for paralysis in thousands of individuals during Prohibition.

Immunosuppression with glucocorticoids is effective in nearly all patients with myasthenia gravis. The therapy presumably works by slowing production of antibodies to the ACh receptors.

130. The answer is D. *(Structure of viruses)* Viruses have either RNA or DNA, not both. Bacteria in the genus *Chlamydia* contain both types of nucleic acid. Both *Chlamydia* and viruses are obligate intracellular parasites, which depend on the host cell for energy. Since some viruses require arthropod vectors, but other viruses (and *Chlamydia*) do not need arthropod vectors, this is not a dependable differentiating characteristic.

131. The answer is C. *(Toxicology)* Benzene is associated with the induction of aplastic anemia by damaging myeloid stem cells. Thiouracil is associated with agranulocytosis, primarily due to its ability to decrease production or increase destruction of neutrophils. Penicillin acts as a hapten, which produces erythrocyte destruction via warm antibody autoimmune hemolysis. In contrast, methyldopa stimulates the production of antibodies against intrinsic red blood cell antigens. Ingestion of an excessive quantity of acetaminophen is followed by the production of toxic metabolites, which first decrease hepatic glutathione levels and then cause a centrolobular necrosis due to biomolecule adduct formation.

132–137. The answers are: 132-C, 133-B, 134-A, 135-E, 136-E, 137-A. *(Exocrine pancreatic function)* Elevated serum amylase is the single most important diagnostic finding for confirmation of acute pancreatitis. A serum amylase level threefold higher than normal virtually confirms the diagnosis.

Secretin is composed of 27 amino acids, is secreted by the mucosal cells of the duodenum, and promotes the secretion of pancreatic juice rich in electrolytes and water.

Cholecystokinin is released by mucosal cells in the upper small intestine in response to peptones and fats. It is absorbed into the bloodstream and stimulates the pancreas to secrete large quantities of digestive enzymes.

Although neuronal control of pancreatic exocrine function is secondary to hormonal control, parasympathetic stimulation of pancreatic secretory activity occurs via vagal fibers, which release acetylcholine (ACh).

Secretin and cholecystokinin are secreted by the mucosa of the small intestine into the bloodstream. They exert their effects after entering the pancreatic circulation. The proteolytic enzymes are synthesized as proenzymes, inactive precursors that must be processed before they are active. Many proenzymes, including chymotrypsinogen, procarboxypeptidase, and prophospholipase, are activated by trypsin. Trypsinogen is activated by enterokinase.

138. The answer is D. *(Cholesterol biosynthesis)* The rate-limiting and regulated step of cholesterol biosynthesis is the formation of mevalonate from β-hydroxy-β-methylglutaryl coenzyme A (HMG CoA) catalyzed by HMG CoA reductase. This enzyme is inhibited by dietary cholesterol and endogenously synthesized cholesterol. A vegetarian diet, a diet low in cholesterol, and the administration of a bile acid–sequestering resin all result in a reduced intake of cholesterol, which will not reduce HMG CoA reductase activity. Familial hypercholesterolemia is a result of a deficiency of low-density lipoprotein (LDL) receptors.

139. The answer is E. *(Bacterial pigment production)* Pseudomonas aeruginosa. Staphylococcus aureus, and Serratia marcescens are all pigment producers. Pigment production by bacteria is associated with both gram-positive and gram-negative organisms. *P. aeruginosa* and *S. marcescens* produce endotoxins, and only *S. aureus* produces enterotoxin and lipoteichoic acids. None of the organisms listed produce mycolic acids.

140 and 141. The answers are: 140-B, 141-A. *(Cardiac dynamics)* The gradient that occurs between the ventricular and aortic systolic pressures is diagnostic of aortic stenosis. The normal aortic valve provides a negligible resistance, and the aortic pressure is nearly identical to the ventricular pressure during the phase of rapid ventricular ejection. A similar picture is seen if right ventricular and pulmonary pressures are measured in the presence of pulmonary valve stenosis, but the pressures are proportionately reduced because of the low resistance of the pulmonary circulation.

Semilunar valve stenosis represents an impediment to the ejection of blood from the ventricle and results in an ejection-type murmur during systole. An ejection murmur is diamond-shaped (i.e., it is a crescendo–decrescendo sound that has maximal intensity in midsystole, when the pressure gradient is largest).

142. The answer is B. *(Genetic code; nucleotides)* Three nucleotides are required to specify the insertion of an amino acid into a polypeptide chain. These groups of three nucleotides comprise a set of codewords that are represented in the 5' to 3' direction. Because there are four different bases in RNA, the maximum number of codons is sixty-four. Sixty-one of these codons specify the twenty amino acids; some amino acids have more than one code word. The triplet AUG also serves as a start signal, and three triplets that do not code for any amino acid serve as stop signals. The genetic code is virtually universal; all organisms use the same codons to translate their genomes into proteins.

143. The answer is D. *(Histamine receptor antagonists)* Cimetidine and ranitidine are H_2-receptor blockers whose main clinical use is in the treatment of ulcers and other peptic disorders. They block the effects of histamine on gastric acid secretion. H_2 antagonists inhibit, not promote, cytochrome P450 enzymes of the liver. H_1 antagonists (diphenhydramine, chlorpheniramine; etc.) are useful in treating allergies. They also have central effects that are useful in preventing motion sickness; however, they can also cause unwanted sedation.

144. The answer is A. *(Collagen biosynthesis)* The biosynthesis of collagen by fibroblasts involves hydroxylation of prolyl and lysyl residues. These reactions are catalyzed by distinct hydroxylases, which require molecular oxygen, α-ketoglutarate, Fe^{2+}, and ascorbate. Hydroxyproline confers stability on the triple helix. Glycosylation occurs by the addition of a disaccharide unit to specific hydroxylysyl residues. By the end of the hydroxylation and glycosylation reactions, the formation of the triple helix is completed and the procollagen molecule is secreted. Following secretion, the globular heads of procollagen are removed from the NH_2- and COOH-terminal regions to produce tropocollagen, which then assembles into collagen fibers.

145. The answer is C. *(Disaccharide structure and function)* The structure shown is that of the milk disaccharide lactose. Lactose is composed of one mole of galactose and one mole of glucose, which are joined by a β-galactosidic linkage. Lactose is the substrate for the intestinal enzyme lactase, which hydrolyzes the disaccharide. Therefore, lactose would not be digested or absorbed by a lactase-deficient child. Since galactosemia arises from an impaired ability to metabolize galactose, lactose would not be a good source of calories for a child with galactosemia. Additional galactose would augment the problem. Since the only requirement for a reducing sugar is an unsubstituted carbonyl group, the disaccharide would give a positive result in the Fehling-Benedict reducing sugar test. The anomeric carbon of the glucose residue is in equilibrium with the open chain structure, thereby providing an unsubstituted carbonyl group.

146. The answer is B. *(Characteristics of chronic type B gastritis)* Chronic type B gastritis is four times more common than type A (fundal) gastritis, the form of chronic gastritis in which there are circulating antibodies to the parietal cells and intrinsic factor. Type B gastritis may result from chronic alcohol or aspirin use, bile reflux, ulcer disease, or postgastrectomy states. Type A is found in elderly individuals and individuals with pernicious anemia. Levels of gastrin tend to be low, and there may be antibodies to gastrin-producing cells in type B gastritis, in contrast to type A gastritis. In type B gastritis, the stomach wall loses its rugal folds and becomes flattened, glazed, and red.

147. The answer is D. *(Cardiac mechanics and sounds)* Pulmonary stenosis and pulmonary hypertension are associated with a prominent S_4 heart sound. Left-to-right shunts involving the left ventricle (e.g., ventricular septal defects and patent ductus arteriosus) are associated with a prominent S_3 heart sound, as are mitral regurgitation and left ventricular failure.

148. The answer is A. *(Embryology of the cardiovascular system)* Both branches of the fourth aortic arch remain intact during fetal development. In adults, the left aortic arch forms the adult aortic arch, and the right aortic arch forms the proximal segment of the right subclavian artery. During development, the first and second aortic arches all but disappear. In adults, they form the maxillary, hyoid, and stapedial arteries. The third aortic arch forms the common carotid artery. The fifth aortic arch disappears. The sixth aortic arch forms the proximal segment of the right pulmonary artery and the ductus arteriosus.

149. The answer is C. *(Antiepileptics)* Phenytoin decreases resting Na^+ flux as well as the flow of Na^+ currents during chemical depolarization or action potential. In the central nervous system (CNS), this results in depression of the generation and transmission of repetitive action potentials in epileptic foci. It is usually the drug of choice for all seizures except absence seizures and, in general, is started alone to assess its efficacy. Phenytoin is associated with potential teratogenic effects (fetal hydantoin syndrome). Other agents like diazepam or phenobarbital affect chloride channels by interacting with gamma-aminobutyrate (GABA) at its receptor site.

150. The answer is C. *(Hemodynamics)* Under the circumstances described in the question, the stroke volume is 100 ml. Cardiac output is the ratio of O_2 consumption to the arteriovenous difference. In this case, it is:

$$\frac{300 \text{ ml/min}}{20 \text{ ml}/100 \text{ ml} - 15 \text{ ml}/100 \text{ ml}} = 6000 \text{ ml/min}$$

Stroke volume is the ratio of cardiac output to heart rate:

$$\frac{6000 \text{ ml/min}}{60 \text{ min}} = 100 \text{ ml}$$

151. The answer is B. *(Gas exchange)* Anemia reduces the oxygen-carrying capacity of the blood but does not affect arterial oxygen tension. Thus, oxygen delivery is decreased and venous oxygen will have a lower partial pressure at rest and during exercise in the anemic subject. The anemic subject is patient B since his oxygen content is reduced for every level of Po_2.

152. The answer is E. *(Pathogenesis of infectious microorganisms)* *Borrelia burgdorferi* is spread by ticks and is the cause of Lyme disease. *Rickettsia rickettsii* also is usually spread by ticks. *Clostridium* *tetani* enters the body through wounds. *Neisseria meningitidis* and *Corynebacterium diphtheriae* both enter via the respiratory tract.

153. The answer is B. *(Gram-negative bacteria)* *Bacillus anthracis* is a gram-positive bacterium and therefore does not produce endotoxin. Endotoxic activity is caused by the lipid A portion of lipopolysaccharide found in the outer membrane of many gram-negative bacteria. *Proteus vulgaris, Escherichia coli, Klebsiella pneumoniae,* and *Serratia marcescens* are all gram-negative bacteria that contain lipopolysaccharide. Because *B. anthracis* is a gram-positive bacterium that does not contain lipopolysaccharide, the antibody mentioned in the question would be ineffective in treating *B. anthracis* infections.

154. The answer is C. *(Etiology of autoimmune disease)* The presence of forbidden clones provides a supply of cells that can recognize self antigens and will serve as cells to stimulate both humoral and cell-mediated immune responses leading to autoimmunity. B-cell deficiency—primarily a lack of circulating B cells—is a primary cause of hypogammaglobulinemia. Type I hypersensitivity (anaphylactic hypersensitivity) is mediated by humoral antibodies, which result from a normal immune response to exogenous antigens. The deletion of forbidden clones leads to tolerance to autoantigens—the opposite of autoimmunity.

155. The answer is A. *(Fatty acids; nutrition)* The only fatty acid in humans that is clearly and unequivocally essential is linoleic acid. If an adequate supply of linoleic acid is provided, arachidonic acid can be synthesized from linoleic acid. Palmitic and decanoic acids can be synthesized de novo by humans. Phytanic acid, which is derived from chlorophyll-containing foods, is toxic if not metabolized. It is metabolized by the α-hydroxylase pathway in peroxisomes.

156. The answer is D. *(Enzyme catalysis)* The rate of an enzyme-catalyzed reaction is inversely proportional to the magnitude of the energy of the transition state. Each enzyme has two characteristic kinetic parameters: V_{max} is an index of the catalytic efficiency, and K_m is a measure of the affinity of the enzyme for the substrate. The binding of substrate to enzyme induces a conformational change in which the functional group that participates in catalysis is appropriately juxtaposed with the substrate bonds that are to be altered in the reaction. General acid–base catalysis is a catalytic mode frequently used by enzymes.

157. The answer is C. *(Anatomy of the respiratory system)* Type II pneumocytes cover less than 5% of the alveolar surface, but they form a reserve for replacement of damaged type I pneumocytes. These multilamellar bodies are the source of the phospholipid-containing pulmonary surfactant. Defects in these cells contribute to infant and adult respiratory distress.

158. The answer is B. *(Gaucher's disease)* Gaucher's disease is a lysosomal storage disease caused by a deficiency of lysosomal β-glucosidase activity. It is an autosomal recessive disease, which is characterized by an absence of glucocerebrosidase with an accumulation of large quantities of β-glucosylceramide in hepatocytes and macrophages. Niemann-Pick disease is characterized by the accumulation of sphingomyelin due to a deficiency in sphingomyelinase. Tay-Sachs disease, in which ganglioside accumulates, results from a lack of N-acetylhexosaminidase. The defective enzyme in gangliosidosis is β-galactosidase.

159. The answer is C. *(Neoplasia of the reproductive tract)* An increased incidence of cancer of the endometrium is associated with obesity, diabetes, hypertension, and infertility; it is not associated with the use of oral contraceptives. Endometrial carcinoma accounts for approximately 7% of invasive cancers in women. It is uncommon in women under age 40 and peaks in incidence between ages 55 and 65.

160. The answer is D. *(Pulmonary mechanics)* Inspiration is an active process brought about by contraction of the diaphragm. This contraction results in increased chest volume, thereby lowering pleural and alveolar pressure and creating a gradient for the movement of air. At the end of inspiration, flow is zero and alveolar pressure equals atmospheric pressure. The difference between alveolar and pleural pressure is the recoil pressure of the lung, which is always greatest at higher lung volumes and thus is greater at the end of inspiration. During expiration, inspiratory muscles relax and the elastic forces of the lungs compress alveolar gas, which raises alveolar pressure to values greater than atmospheric pressure and creates a pressure gradient to expel gas from the lung.

161–165. The answers are: 161-A, 162-B, 163-D, 164-A, 165-C. *(Vitamin deficiency)* Pellagra, a disease affecting the skin (dermatitis), the gastrointestinal tract (diarrhea), and the central nervous system (CNS) [dementia], is the result of a niacin deficiency. Because niacin can be formed from tryptophan, an essential amino acid, dietary treatment of pellagra must take into consideration daily allowances for both niacin and tryptophan. Endemic pellagra is no longer a common occurrence; however, it is a manifestation of two disorders of tryptophan metabolism, Hartnup disease and the carcinoid syndrome. Hartnup disease is an autosomal recessive defect in which patients have a reduced ability to convert tryptophan to niacin. In the carcinoid syndrome, dietary tryptophan is metabolized in the hydroxylation pathway (a minor pathway), leaving little tryptophan for the formation of niacin. Administration of large amounts of niacin can cure the pellagra associated with these conditions.

Beriberi is a severe thiamine deficiency syndrome associated with malnutrition endemic to areas where there is a high intake of highly milled (polished) rice. Clinical characteristics of this deficiency range from cardiovascular and neurologic lesions to emotional disturbances. Cardiovascular changes include right-sided enlargement (dilatation), tachycardia, and "high-output" cardiac failure. Neuromuscular manifestations include peripheral neuropathy (neuritis), weakness, fatigue, and an impaired capacity to do work. Edema and anorexia are also characteristic. In the United States, thiamine deficiency is seen primarily in association with chronic alcoholism, which leads to Wernicke's encephalopathy, which presents with the classic triad of confusion, ataxia, and ophthalmoplegia. In thiamine deficiency, motor and sensory peripheral nerve lesions are marked by neuromuscular findings of numbness and tingling of the legs, and atrophy and weakness of the muscles of the extremities compounded by the loss of reflexes. Mental depression may also accompany these findings. The dementia caused by niacin deficiency results from degeneration of the ganglion cells of the brain, accompanied by degeneration of the fibers of the spinal cord.

166–170. The answers are: 166-E, 167-A, 168-B, 169-D, 170-C. *(Endocrine syndromes)* Bartter's syndrome is a form of secondary hyperaldosteronism in which excessive renin production occurs. The hyperreninemia results from hyperplasia of renal juxtaglomerular cells, which secrete renin primarily in response to decreased arterial blood pressure in afferent arterioles and increased renal sympathetic nerve activity.

Sheehan's syndrome, or postpartum pituitary necrosis, results from the infarction of the anterior lobe of the pituitary gland. Sheehan's syndrome usually is precipitated by obstetric hemorrhage or shock; however, it also can occur in nonpregnant women as well as in men. The infarct usually causes the destruction of 95% to 99% of the anterior lobe.

Cushing's syndrome is characterized by a prolonged overproduction of cortisol. The pituitary gland regulates the synthesis of adrenal cortisol by secreting adrenocorticotropic hormone (ACTH). The secretion of ACTH is regulated by corticotropin-releasing hormone (CRH), which is produced in the hypothalamus. Possible causes of Cushing's syndrome include: ACTH-producing pituitary neoplasm; CRH-producing hypothalamic neoplasm; adrenal cortex cortisol-producing neoplasm; and ectopic ACTH- or CRH-producing neoplasm. Cushing's syndrome can be caused iatrogenically by long-term glucocorticoid therapy.

Waterhouse-Friderichsen syndrome is most often caused by meningococcemia and is characterized by extensive cutaneous petechiae, purpura, and hemorrhages. Skin lesions appear shortly after the onset of an infectious febrile reaction, and the patient may go into circulatory collapse and die within 24 hours. In addition to lesions, extensive internal hemorrhages are present, particularly in the adrenal glands.

Conn's syndrome, or primary hyperaldosteronism, is associated with hypernatremia, hypokalemia, alkalosis, potassium wasting, and low levels of renin.

171–175. The answers are: 171-A, 172-D, 173-E, 174-C, 175-B. *(Cranial vasculature)* The foramen spinosum transmits the middle meningeal artery (A), a branch of the maxillary artery. The carotid canal (D) transmits the internal carotid artery, while the jugular foramen (E) contains the internal jugular vein in addition to the glossopharyngeal, vagus, and spinal accessory nerves. Each posterior condylar canal (C) transmits a large emissary vein. The vertebral arteries enter the cranial cavity through the foramen magnum (B) along with the spinal accessory nerve; the spinal cord also transits the foramen magnum.

176–180. The answers are: 176-A, 177-D, 178-C, 179-B, 180-E. *(Systemic blood pressure)* Normal blood pressure is 140/90 or less in adults. If only the systolic pressure is elevated, this is called isolated systolic hypertension; if the word "hypertension" is used without further qualification, it is presumed that both the systolic and the diastolic elements are high. The normal response to standing upright is a slight rise in pulse rate, a small drop in systolic pressure, and a small rise in diastolic pressure. With volume depletion, both the systolic and the diastolic pressure often drop more considerably; however, if the host has intact vascular reflexes, the pressures may be maintained, or nearly so, by a marked increase in heart rate. This is the situation depicted in the 59-year-old man, where the pressures are almost steady, but at the cost of a 23-beat rise in heart rate. If the pressures drop and there is no compensatory increase in heart rate, the autonomic response is dysfunctional, as shown in the 68-year-old man.

181–185. The answers are: 181-E, 182-D, 183-C, 184-B, 185-A. *(Lipoproteins and genetic disorders)* Lipoprotein lipase is an enzyme normally located within the capillary endothelium; it is involved in converting chylomicrons to chylomicron remnants. Chylomicron levels may also be elevated in systemic lupus erythematosus (SLE).

Familial hypercholesterolemia, due to mutation within a single gene, is one of the most common human mendelian disorders. Low-density lipoprotein (LDL) levels are elevated in the serum because this disorder markedly decreases the number of high-affinity LDL receptors within the liver. LDL levels may also be elevated in nephrotic syndrome and hyperthyroidism.

Familial (type III) hyperlipoproteinemia has been traced to a single amino acid substitution within the receptor for apoprotein E. As the apoprotein E receptor is required for the normal metabolism of both chylomicron remnants and intermediate-density lipoproteins, both of these molecules accumulate in the blood.

The biochemical defect underlying familial hypertriglyceridemia is unknown. In this disorder, serum levels of both very low-density lipoprotein (VLDL) and triglycerides are elevated. VLDL and triglyceride levels may also be elevated in diabetes mellitus and chronic alcoholism.

The defect underlying familial hyperlipidemia is unknown, although research suggests a deficiency in apoprotein CII. In this disorder, serum levels of VLDL and chylomicrons are elevated; alcoholism, diabetes mellitus, and oral contraceptives are also capable of elevating VLDL and chylomicron levels.

186–191. The answers are: 186-A, 187-C, 188-B, 189-F, 190-E, 191-D. *(Gross and microscopic appearances of neoplasms)* Grossly, the squamous cell carcinoma is a firm, white–tan mass, approximately 2 cm in diameter. Histologically, the neoplasm displays nuclei having hyperchromatic coarse chromatin; nucleoli may or may not be observed. The tumor may be indolent, with a prominent host response consisting of inflammation and fibroblastic proliferation.

Grossly, the bronchioalveolar adenocarcinoma is white and granular and ranges from several millimeters to several centimeters in diameter. On chest x-ray, the lesion may resemble "fluffy" infiltrates of pneumonia. This tumor also follows a rather indolent course, but the multicentric foci, which appear to result from aerogenic spread, limit resectability.

Grossly, the type of adenocarcinoma usually seen often appears as a tan mass between 1 cm and 3 cm in diameter. Histologically, the tumor cell cytoplasm is pale-staining and may contain mucin vacuoles. The nuclei are round or oval, with delicate chromatin patterns and prominent nucleoli. This tumor often metastasizes early to the brain.

Grossly, carcinoid often appears as a fleshy, brown, intrabronchial polyp. Histologically, the tumor grows in a pattern of clusters or ribbons of cells. The neurosecretory granules may contain neuron-specific enolase, bombesin, serotonin, calcitonin, gastrin, adrenocorticotropic hormone (ACTH), and somatostatin, among other materials. A carcinoid often arises in the appendix and terminal ileum.

The rapidly replicating small, primitive-appearing cells of small cell (oat cell) carcinoma have finely stippled nuclei, a high nuclear:cytoplasm ratio, and nucleoli that are not prominent. The small, dense neurosecretory granules may contain markers such as neuron-specific enolase, bombesin, calcitonin, somatostatin, vasoactive intestinal polypeptide (VIP), or ACTH. Long-term survival is poor due to extensive metastases to the liver, brain, bone, or adrenal glands by the time of diagnosis.

The large cell carcinoma is usually 3 cm to 6 cm in diameter. It is a white–tan tumor that is partially necrotic or cavitating. In addition to the leukemoid reaction, the presence of this tumor may also be manifested by elevated serum levels of the β-chain of chorionic gonadotropin.

192–194. The answers are: 192-C, 193-A, 194-B. *(Hepatic histology)* This is a scanning electron micrograph of the liver. Liver parenchymal cells (A) secrete bile into the bile canaliculi (B) and blood proteins, such as serum albumin and transferrin, into the liver sinusoids (C). Liver sinusoids are modified fenestrated and discontinuous capillaries that receive blood from the portal vein and hepatic artery in the portal canals and carry it to the central veins.

195–199. The answers are: 195-A, 196-B, 197-A, 198-B, 199-B. *(Myocardial infarction)* As time passes after a myocardial infarction, the morphologic features vary. Six hours after the acute event, the gross appearance of the myocardium is normal. However, visible gross changes can be seen 18 to 24 hours postinfarction, such as pallor of the myocardium. Increased serum levels of creatinine kinase and lactate dehydrogenase can aid in the diagnosis if measurements are taken within 1 to 3 days. Electrocardiographic disturbances can be seen immediately. Although histologic signs can be seen within 12 hours postinfarction, peak neutrophil infiltration cannot be seen for 1 to 3 days. Maximal coagulative necrosis can be seen 24 to 72 hours postinfarction, after which time macrophages destroy the necrotic myocytes.

200–204. The answers are: 200-D, 201-B, 202-C, 203-C, 204-B. *(Embryology)* Ectoderm gives rise to the nervous system, sensory epithelia, epidermis, mammary glands, and the pituitary gland. Melanocytes in the dermis arise from neuroectoderm. Mesoderm gives rise to cartilage, bone, connective tissue, muscles, the cardiovascular system, kidneys, gonads, spleen, and the adrenal cortex. Endoderm gives rise to gastrointestinal and respiratory mucosa, and the parenchyma of the tonsils, thyroid gland, parathyroid glands, thymus, liver, and pancreas.

205–207. The answers are: 205-C, 206-B, 207-B. *(Anatomy of abdominal fascia)* The abdominal superficial fascia (subcutaneous tissue) has two layers: The superficial fatty layer is called Camper's fascia; the deep membranous layer is called Scarpa's fascia. Both are especially prominent over the abdominal wall. Of these two layers, only Scarpa's fascia can support sutures. Scarpa's fascia continues over the pubis and perineum as Colles' fascia.

208–212. The answers are: 208-C, 209-A, 210-E, 211-B, 212-D. *(Placental anatomy)* The placenta consists of a decidual plate (C) facing the endometrium and a chorionic plate (E) facing the fetus. The decidual plate and chorionic plate are fused at the margins of the discoid placenta. These two plates are interconnected by cytotrophoblastic cell columns (B). Large numbers of chorionic villi (D) project away from them into the intervillous space (A). Maternal blood vessels end on the decidual plate and pour maternal blood into the intervillous space. Maternal blood directly bathes the chorionic villi. Thus, the human placenta is said to be a hemochorial placenta.

213–217. The answers are: 213-B, 214-C, 215-A, 216-D, 217-E. *(Neuroanatomy)* Many neuroanatomical pathways now can be specified by their neurotransmitters. Thus, selective depletion of the neurotransmitters can be caused by sectioning the pathways or by destroying the perikarya that produce the neurotransmitter.

Destruction of interneurons of the spinal cord would deplete gamma-aminobutyric acid (GABA) and glycine, inhibitory transmitters produced by interneurons. Section of the medial forebrain bundle would destroy many of the axons that connect the catecholaminergic and serotoninergic nuclei of the brain stem with the cerebral cortex. Destruction of the medullary raphe would destroy the serotoninergic neurons of the medulla that project to the spinal cord. Dorsal root section would reduce substance P concentration in the dorsal horns. This neurotransmitter presumably transmits pain impulses from the small fibers in the lateral division of the dorsal roots.

Not only can the neurotransmitters be depleted by actual anatomical destruction of axonal pathways or the destruction of neuronal perikarya, but various drugs and chemicals can also selectively block neurotransmitters either by inhibiting their formation, inhibiting their release, or competing with binding sites on the postsynaptic membrane. By combining anatomical lesions with chemical blockade and direct chemical analysis, various lines of evidence can be developed to establish the transmitters involved in the various layers and regions of the cortex and the different nuclei of the central nervous system (CNS).

218–222. The answers are: 218-F, 219-D, 220-A, 221-E, 222-C. *(Tumors of the musculoskeletal system)* A chondroblastoma is a benign tumor composed of small immature chondrocytes, each with a single nucleus, dispersed among benign-appearing, multinucleated giant cells and chondroid matrix. This tumor most often occurs within the epiphyseal region of long, tubular bones of individuals between the ages of 10 and 20 years. Males are affected twice as often as females.

A giant cell tumor is a benign, but locally invasive, lesion characterized by many multinucleated giant cells distributed in a stroma of neoplastic, smaller, mononucleated cells. Over 50% of these "brown" tumors develop in the distal femur or proximal tibia or fibula. The majority of individuals with this tumor are between 20 and 40 years of age. Females are affected slightly more often than males. The tumor frequently recurs many years after surgical removal.

An osteosarcoma is a malignant tumor that most often arises in the medullary cavity of the metaphyseal end of the long bones of the extremities. It is a tumor of mesenchymal cells in which there is deposition of osteoid or new bone. This tumor is most often seen in adolescent or young adult males. Deletions of the long arm of chromosome 13, which are associated with retinoblastoma, are hypothesized to be associated with osteosarcoma development. Radiographs of osteosarcomas often visualize Codman's triangle—an angle formed between the elevated periosteum and the plane of the outer surface of the cortical bone.

Osteoid osteoma is a small, extremely painful benign tumor without the potential for malignant transformation. Radiographically, it appears as small, radiolucent foci surrounded by dense sclerotic bone. Most lesions are intracortical and arise near the ends of the femur or tibia. The lesion appears most often in individuals between 5 and 25 years of age, and it occurs twice as often in males as in females.

Ewing's sarcoma is a malignant neoplasm, most often seen in the pelvis and long tubular bones. It is characterized radiographically by "onion-skin" layering of the cortex and widening of the diaphyseal region. Ewing's sarcoma usually arises before the age of 20 years, and it appears twice as often in males as in females. This tumor is associated with translocation of portions of the long arms of chromosomes 11 and 22. The majority of chondrosarcomas affect the pelvis and ribs; they most often occur between the middle and the end of the life span.

223–228. The answers are: 223-E, 224-A, 225-C, 226-A, 227-D, 228-B. *(Etiology of spirochetal diseases) Borrelia recurrentis* is the etiologic agent of relapsing fever in humans. The disease occurs worldwide and is characterized by a febrile bacteremia. The disease name is derived from the fact that 3 to 10 recurrences can occur, apparently from the original infection. The disease is transmitted to humans from infected animals by ticks and from human to human by lice.

Bejel is nonvenereal, endemic syphilis caused by a variant of *Treponema pallidum*. The disease usually is seen in children in the Middle East and Africa. Transmission appears to be through the shared use of drinking and eating utensils; bejel is not transmitted sexually. The disease develops in primary, secondary, and tertiary stages.

Pinta is a tropical disease caused by *Treponema carateum*. It occurs primarily in Central and South America, where it appears to be spread by person-to-person contact. Unlike other treponemal diseases, the lesions of pinta remain localized in the skin.

The etiologic agent of syphilis is *T. pallidum*. Humans are the only natural host of the spirochete, and venereal transmission is the most common means of acquiring the infection. Congenital syphilis occurs when the fetus is infected transplacentally and survives to delivery. Accidental laboratory infections occasionally occur.

Fort Bragg fever is a localized name of pretibial fever caused by *Leptospira interrogans* serogroup *autumnalis*. The disease is characterized by a rash on the shins. Humans probably acquire the infection by contact with the urine of infected animals.

Treponema pertenue is the etiologic agent of yaws. The disease occurs primarily in children in tropical regions, where it appears to be transmitted by direct contact or by vectors such as flies. This potentially disfiguring disease has primary, secondary, and tertiary stages.

229–232. The answers are: 229-C, 230-A, 231-D, 232-E. *(Neurophysiology and visual science)* Presbyopia (impairment of vision due to old age) is caused by a decrease in the elasticity of the lens. As a result, the eyes are unable to accommodate for near vision. Another condition associated with aging is cataracts, in which the lens becomes progressively less transparent. Myopia is caused by an overall refractive power that is too great for the axial length of the eyeball. It causes distant objects to be focused in front of the retina and can be corrected by a diverging lens. In hyperopia, the overall refractive power is too low for the axial length of the eyeball, and so the eyes must continuously accommodate to see distant objects clearly.

233–237. The answers are: 233-B, 234-D, 235-E, 236-A, 237-C. *(Transport proteins)* The functions of transport proteins can be divided into three general classes: the control of diffusion into the tissues; the highly specific recognition of molecules; and the removal of toxins. Transferrin helps in transporting iron to storage and utilization sites in the bone marrow. The damage that free iron can cause to tissues other than the marrow is prevented when it is bound by transferrin. Transcobalamin binds vitamin B_{12} and prevents it from degrading while it is being transported to storage and utilization sites in tissues with high cellular turnover rates. Albumin is the main plasma protein responsible for the maintenance of serum osmotic pressure. Haptoglobin is a plasma protein that binds free hemoglobin in the blood and delivers it to the liver for recycling. The degree of intravascular hemolysis is determined by measuring the levels of depleted free forms of haptoglobin in the blood.

238–243. The answers are: 238-A, 239-C, 240-B, 241-B, 242-A, 243-A. *(Abnormal heart sounds)* The first heart sound, S_1, is composed of the sounds of tricuspid and mitral valve closure. Mitral valve closure is normally almost silent, and S_1 is normally quieter than the second heart sound, S_2, which is the sound of the aortic and pulmonic valves closing. S_1 is better heard at the apex of the heart, and S_2 is better heard at the base of the heart. With mitral valve stenosis, the left ventricle is underfilled at the end of diastole, and its systolic contraction has force sufficient to cause the mitral valve leaflets to close audibly. During ventricular systole, the presence of aortic stenosis produces a high flow rate through the stenotic valve, which is appreciated as a pansystolic murmur. The sound is heard well at both the base and apex of the heart and is relatively unchanged by respiratory movements. In acute aortic regurgitation, the left ventricle is overfilled and the ejection fraction is reduced. During ventricular systole, the pressure buildup is more sluggish than normal due to the leaking aortic valve. The mitral valve closure becomes even quieter than normal; thus, S_1 is quieter than normal. In systemic hypertension, the higher than normal pressure within the aortic bulb at the end of systole causes the very forceful closure of the aortic valve, which produces an S_2 that is louder than usual. In cases of severe anemia or hyperthyroidism, the heart rate is increased along with cardiac output. The increase in heart rate causes the heart to spend a greater portion of its time in systole and less time in diastole. The reduction in diastolic time means that the left ventricle may be relatively underfilled at the beginning of systole. As stated above, the contraction of an underfilled ventricle allows the mitral valve to close with force sufficient to cause S_1 to be louder than S_2.

244–247. The answers are: 244-A, 245-C, 246-B, 247-A. *(Pelvic innervation)* Afferent nerves from the pelvic viscera travel along autonomic pathways. Afferents from the ovary, testis, upper to middle ureter, uterine tubes, urinary bladder, and uterine body travel along the least splanchnic nerve to the lower thoracic segment and along the lumbar splanchnic nerves to the upper lumbar segments of the spinal cord; thus, pain is referred to the inguinal and pubic regions as well as the lateral and anterior aspects of the thigh. Afferents from the epididymis, uterine cervix, and distal ureter travel along the pelvic splanchnic nerves to the midsacral spinal segments; thus, pain is referred to the perineum, posterior thigh, and leg.

248–250. The answers are: 248-B, 249-A, 250-D. *(Inflammatory heart disease)* Chronic rheumatic heart disease refers to the long-term cardiac complications (especially valvular) of acute rheumatic fever. Typically, the mitral and aortic valve leaflets become thickened and deformed by fibrosis, with commissural fusion. The damaged valves represent a fertile ground for the development of infective endocarditis (subacute type).

Chronic rheumatic heart disease is a complication of acute rheumatic fever, which is a nonsuppurative systemic disorder related to an untreated pharyngitis caused by group A β-hemolytic streptococci. Although the precise mechanism of acute rheumatic fever is unknown, the presence of antistreptococcal antibodies that cross-react with heart antigens in these patients suggests an autoimmune basis for this disorder.

Subacute bacterial endocarditis most commonly is caused by α-hemolytic (viridans) streptococci, organisms that are a normal component of the oral flora. Typically, the organism gains entry to the circulation with minor oral trauma, and a transient bacteremia ensues. The bacteria then colonize a platelet-fibrin thrombus that has formed on a valve previously damaged by chronic rheumatic heart disease, mitral valve prolapse, previous cardiac surgery, or some other cause.

The acute form of bacterial endocarditis, in contrast to the subacute form, typically involves a normal heart valve in the setting of a well-defined bacteremia. In this case, the infectious agent usually is a virulent organism (e.g., *Staphylococcus aureus*) that causes the initial damage to the valves by way of a toxin.

Libman-Sacks endocarditis (also known as nonbacterial verrucous endocarditis) may occur as a complication of systemic lupus erythematosus (SLE). This disorder is characterized by the presence of warty endocardial vegetations along the valve margins and, most distinctively, on the undersurface of the valves.

Practice Examination II

QUESTIONS

Directions: Each of the numbered items or incomplete statements in this section is followed by answers or by completions of the statement. Select the **one** lettered answer or completion that is **best** in each case.

1. A correct description of the individual curves depicted in the log–dose response relationship below includes which of the following?

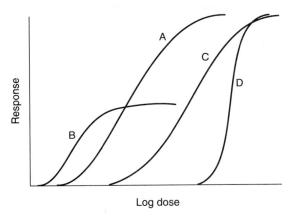

(A) curves A and D: a full agonist (drug A) and a partial agonist (drug D)
(B) curves B and C: an agonist in the absence of a noncompetitive inhibitor (curve B) and in the presence of one (curve C)
(C) curves A, C, and D: three agonists with similar efficacy but different potency
(D) curves A and C: an agonist in the absence of a competitive inhibitor (curve C) and in the presence of one (curve A)
(E) curves A and C: drug A is less potent than drug C

2. Androgens are not only important hormones in male reproductive physiology but also are currently an abused group of agents for presumptive improvement of athletic prowess. Exogenous administration of large amounts of testosterone is likely to produce all of the following effects EXCEPT

(A) masculinization in mature females
(B) feminization in mature males
(C) closure of the epiphyses of long bones
(D) an increase in sperm count

3. A 25-year-old man is admitted to the surgery unit for arthroscopic examination of his left knee. After discussion with the anesthesiologist, the patient elects to have a spinal anesthetic. Which of the following anatomic landmarks are relevant for obtaining access to the intrathecal space?

(A) Midline between T10 and T11
(B) Paramedian between C5 and C6
(C) L3–L4 at the level of the iliac crest
(D) Anterior at the level of the stellate ganglion
(E) The sacral hiatus between S3 and S5

4. A patient is on a ventilator. The patient's anatomic dead space is 150 ml and the ventilator's dead space is 250 ml. The ventilatory rate is set at 20 times per minute. What should the output (tidal volume) of the ventilator be adjusted to so that alveolar minute ventilation is 4 L/min?

(A) 150 ml
(B) 250 ml
(C) 400 ml
(D) 600 ml
(E) 1000 ml

5. Angiotensin-converting enzyme (ACE) hydrolyzes angiotensin I to angiotensin II. Possible explanations why inhibition of this enzyme with specific peptide inhibitors (i.e., captopril) reduces blood pressure in some subjects include all of the following EXCEPT

(A) decreased production of a vasoconstrictor (angiotensin II)
(B) increased synthesis and release of aldosterone
(C) centrally mediated decrease in water intake
(D) inhibition of synaptic transmission in peripheral sympathetic nervous system

Questions 6–8

A physician who has recommended urography for her competent, 68-year-old male patient is trying to decide whether or not to disclose the remote risk (1 in 10,000) of a fatal reaction.

6. If the physician favors nondisclosure, reasoning that it would not be in the patient's best interests to worry him with such remote risks, the physician is guided by

(A) beneficence but not nonmaleficence
(B) nonmaleficence but not beneficence
(C) both beneficence and nonmaleficence
(D) justice
(E) gratitude

7. If the physician believes that her decision should be determined by what other physicians would do in similar circumstances, she is guided by

(A) both beneficence and nonmaleficence
(B) strong paternalism
(C) weak paternalism
(D) respect for autonomy
(E) the professional practice standard

8. If the physician bases her decision on her assessment of whether or not the patient would want to learn about such remote risks, the physician is guided by

(A) respect for autonomy
(B) beneficence
(C) nonmaleficence
(D) both beneficence and nonmaleficence
(E) the professional practice standard

9. Correct statements concerning toxic exposure to organophosphates include which one of the following?

(A) Aminophylline is the agent of first choice in reversing the respiratory symptoms
(B) Atropine and pralidoxime are useful antidotes
(C) Exposure must be inhalational since organophosphates are not well-absorbed through the skin
(D) Immediate injection of epinephrine is a useful antidote

Questions 10–13

A new resident at a teaching hospital examines a 46-year-old man who presents with abdominal pain, diarrhea, and arthralgia. A history and physical examination reveal progressive weight loss, low-grade fever, peripheral lymphadenopathy, and borderline anemia.

10. The resident should order all of the following laboratory tests at this time EXCEPT

(A) xylose absorption
(B) small bowel x-rays
(C) oral [^{14}C]triolein for stool fat
(D) serum gastrin levels
(E) endoscopic retrograde cholangiopancreatography (ERCP)

11. The serum gastrin level is within the normal range. However, jejunal biopsy reveals dilated lacteals and the presence of numerous mucosal macrophages containing large cytoplasmic granules staining with periodic acid–Schiff reagent. Based on these data, a working diagnosis is

(A) liver and biliary tract disease
(B) Zollinger-Ellison syndrome
(C) amyloidosis
(D) Whipple's disease
(E) agammaglobulinemia

12. The laboratory test results are consistent with the diagnosis, and the resident handling this case is congratulated by the chief resident for her clinical acumen. The treatment of choice is now

(A) fat-restricted diet and vitamin supplementation
(B) trimethoprim-sulfamethoxazole
(C) prednisone/melphalan/colchicine
(D) cholestyramine
(E) cimetidine or another H_2-receptor antagonist

13. The patient may also do well if the primary therapy is supplemented for a short time with

(A) vitamins D and K
(B) gamma globulin (IgG)
(C) cyanocobalamin
(D) omeprazole
(E) cimetidine and fluids

14. Of the following statements regarding thoracic outlet syndrome, which one is true?

(A) It results from an irregularly shaped first thoracic rib
(B) Compression of the left phrenic nerve may occur
(C) Numbness and tingling occur along a median nerve distribution
(D) Compression of the subclavian artery may occur

15. A patient has a lifelong history of bruising and is now scheduled for elective hernia repair. He has no other medical problems and is taking no medications. The bleeding time is two to three times normal. The platelet count and all other screening coagulation tests are normal. Review of the peripheral smear is unremarkable. The next step to take for this patient is to

(A) perform antiplatelet antibody detection tests
(B) perform platelet aggregation studies
(C) proceed with surgery as planned
(D) proceed with surgery after transfusion with platelets
(E) proceed with surgery after treatment with 1-desamino-8-D-arginine vasopressin (DDAVP)

16. A 42-year-old woman with breast cancer was treated with irradiation and currently is receiving chemotherapy. She complained of some left-sided chest pain, which was determined not to be of cardiac origin. On the fourth day, several vesicles appeared on her left thorax, following a rib in distribution; she also had several smaller vesicles at other sites (scalp, leg, forearm). Her physician diagnosed varicella–zoster virus (VZV) infection and started treatment with acyclovir. Which one of the following statements best describes the VZV in this case?

(A) Thymidine kinase–negative VZV mutants are likely to render the treatment ineffective
(B) The initial exposure to VZV in childhood could not have led to viral latency in the dorsal ganglia
(C) The lesions outside the dermatomal distribution are likely explained by depressed cell-mediated immunity

17. In patients with Barrett's esophagus, factors responsible for the morphologic changes in the distal portion of the esophagus from normal squamous cell epithelium to columnar epithelium include all of the following EXCEPT

(A) incompetence of the lower esophageal sphincter
(B) the ingrowth of immature pluripotent stem cells
(C) increased exposure to acid and pepsin
(D) the absence of inflammatory processes
(E) increased exposure to bile acids and lysolecithin

18. The role of a viral envelope primarily is that it

(A) gives the virus particle greater resistance to unfavorable environmental conditions
(B) interacts and thus stabilizes the viral genome
(C) contains those virus proteins that recognize receptors on susceptible cells
(D) allows the virus particle to fuse with cellular membranes, thus bypassing the requirement of viral protein–cell receptor interactions

19. Specific and significant toxicities are often associated with the use of antineoplastic agents. An important dose-limiting effect on the kidney is associated with which one of the following antineoplastic agents?

(A) Bleomycin
(B) Busulfan
(C) Cisplatin
(D) Methotrexate
(E) Vincristine

20. The female reproductive viscera are best characterized by which of the following statements?

(A) The mesosalpinx contains the tubal branches of the uterine vessels
(B) The ovarian veins drain directly into the inferior vena cava
(C) Lymph from the cervix drains into the inguinal nodes
(D) Visceral afferent nerves from the body of the uterus course along the pelvic splanchnic nerves

21. An increase in plasma Na⁺ concentrations (hypernatremia) with normal blood volumes causes which one of the following actions?

(A) Release of antidiuretic hormone from the posterior pituitary
(B) Release of aldosterone from the adrenal gland
(C) Release of renin from the juxtaglomerular cells
(D) Decrease in renal excretion of Na⁺

Questions 22 and 23

Cystic fibrosis (CF) is an autosomal recessive disease with an incidence of 1 per 1600 in the Caucasian population.

22. What is the frequency of the cystic fibrosis gene?

(A) 1/4
(B) 1/20
(C) 1/40
(D) 1/200
(E) 1/400

23. Of the following values, what proportion of the nomal siblings of CF individuals would most likely be carriers?

(A) 1/4
(B) 1/2
(C) 2/3
(D) All
(E) None

Questions 24 and 25

A pregnant Iraqi refugee presents for prenatal care. Remembering the high incidence of various infectious diseases due to the war, the physician is especially thorough in his examination. The history includes a period of jaundice accompanied by intestinal upset and serum sickness–associated symptoms 3 years prior to her pregnancy. The physician considers the possibility of chronic hepatitis in this patient and the possible threat to her newborn as a result of a perinatal infection.

24. The etiologic agent that the physician should be most concerned about in this case is

(A) hepatitis A virus
(B) hepatitis B virus
(C) Epstein-Barr virus
(D) delta hepatitis virus
(E) cytomegalovirus

25. Which one of the following laboratory tests should be ordered to aid in the diagnosis of the maternal infection?

(A) Tests for acute and convalescent cytomegalovirus complement-fixing antibody levels
(B) Quantitation of the hepatitis A virus IgM antibody
(C) Tests for hepatitis B virus surface antigen (HBsAg) and HBeAg, as well as for antibody to HBsAg

26. Diabetes mellitus is a major cause of renal disease and mortality. Several key features of diabetes mellitus–associated renal pathology include all of the following EXCEPT

(A) capillary basement membrane thickening
(B) infiltration of glomeruli with leukocytes and monocytes
(C) diffuse glomerulosclerosis
(D) nodular glomerulosclerosis

Questions 27–29

A female infant is to be evaluated for developmental impairment, short stature, and unusual facial features. In addition to short stature, examination reveals small head circumference, flattened facial features, epicanthal folds, upslanted palpebral fissures, protuberant tongue, excessive nuchal skin, bilateral simian creases, and generalized hypotonia.

27. The best method for diagnosing this condition is

(A) developmental assessment
(B) karyotype
(C) electroencephalogram
(D) urine spot test for mucopolysaccharides

28. How does this clinical condition arise?

(A) Radiation exposure during pregnancy
(B) Drug exposure during pregnancy
(C) Nondisjunction
(D) None of the above

29. The parents are planning to have another child. What is the risk that this condition will occur again?

(A) 1 in 4
(B) 2 in 4
(C) 1 in 100
(D) Not estimable

Questions 30–35

A 48-year-old woman, with no previous history of heart disease or angina pectoris, is diagnosed as having stage III ovarian carcinoma. After a surgical procedure to remove the bulk of her tumor, she is given anticancer chemotherapy. Months later she is admitted to the hospital for a follow-up laparotomy. She is given cefoxitin intravenously and 10 minutes later develops severe hypotension with systolic blood pressure of 40 to 50 mm Hg, wheezing, and urticaria. The laparotomy is postponed, and the patient is given intravenous epinephrine, dexamethasone, diphenhydramine, and fluids. After restoration of normal blood pressure, an electrocardiograph suggests acute cardiac injury. Subsequent chest x-ray reveals a normal heart size with bilateral pulmonary edema.

30. All of the following are anticancer agents EXCEPT

(A) adriamycin
(B) gentamicin
(C) cisplatin
(D) cyclophosphamide
(E) melphalan

31. Which one of the following was the rationale for the administration of cefoxitin in the above patient? It

(A) is selectively distributed into the peritoneal cavity, the site of the surgery
(B) can be administered orally if necessary
(C) has some intrinsic antineoplastic activity
(D) is effective against gram-negative and gram-positive organisms
(E) can be administered simultaneously with aminoglycosides

32. The most likely cause of the hypotension, urticaria, and wheezing seen in this patient might be a

(A) type I IgE-mediated allergic response
(B) type II IgM and IgG cytolytic allergic response
(C) type III IgG complement-mediated inflammatory response
(D) type IV cellular hypersensitivity response
(E) type V IgA cytokine-mediated response

33. What is the underlying mechanism for the woman's immunologic response?

(A) Complement-mediated injury involving soluble antibodies and any cell with isoantigen
(B) Complement–mediated inflammatory response initiated by soluble antigen–antibody complexes
(C) Lymphokine-induced injury to macrophages and lymphocytes
(D) Cytolytic injury due to sensitized lymphocytes and macrophages
(E) Release of noncytolytic mediators from basophilic leukocytes and tissue mast cells

34. The pharmacologic reasons for administering epinephrine, dexamethasone, and diphenhydramine include all of the following EXCEPT to

(A) block the release of endogenous mediators
(B) competitively block endogenous receptors of the response
(C) decrease capillary permeability
(D) induce bronchoconstriction
(E) inhibit cellular proliferation

35. What is the likely physiologic basis for the cardiovascular changes in this patient?

(A) Sensitization of the heart to antibody–antigen complexes and transient hypoxia-mediated cardiac effects
(B) Infiltration of lymphocytes, neutrophils, and mast cells into the heart tissue
(C) Direct toxicity to and electrophysiologic pertubations in the His–Purkinje system by cefoxitin
(D) Acute vasoconstriction in the left circumflex and right coronary arteries
(E) Parasympathetic nervous system (vagal) activation mediated by direct effects of cefoxitin

36. Hodgkin's lymphoma can be distinguished from other forms of lymphoma by the presence of

(A) Reed-Sternberg cells
(B) the Philadelphia chromosome
(C) Auer rods
(D) decreased quantities of leukocyte alkaline phosphatase

37. A patient injected with horse anti–rattlesnake venom serum complains of general weakness, headaches, and muscle and joint pains. He notices that his urine is darker 10 days after the injection. A urine test shows increased elimination of proteins. Laboratory tests show normal immunoglobulin levels and low serum C4 and C3 levels. The most likely cause of this clinical situation is

(A) a systemic reaction to snake venom released after the effects of the antitoxin have disappeared
(B) deposition of antigen–antibody complexes made of snake venom proteins and horse antibody
(C) delayed hypersensitivity to horse proteins
(D) an anaphylactic reaction (type I) to snake venom
(E) deposition of antigen–antibody complexes made of horse proteins and human immunoglobulins

38. A patient with a metastatic melanoma was treated with a mouse monoclonal antibody that was specific for the tumor-associated antigen and capable of lysing the malignant cells in vitro with complement addition. A partial reduction of the tumor mass was achieved during the early part of the treatment. Then the patient showed increased numbers of metastases to new sites, including the liver, in spite of increased amounts and more frequent injections of the monoclonal antibody. All of the following factors explain the problem EXCEPT

(A) mutation of the tumor-associated antigen gene
(B) complement depletion as a result of the liver metastasis
(C) appearance of antibodies to mouse immunoglobulins
(D) low blood levels of soluble tumor-associated antigen

39. Which of the following statements concerning acetylsalicylic acid (aspirin), the prototype of a group of nonsteroidal anti-inflammatory agents that are also analgesic and antipyretic, is correct?

(A) Aspirin is a potent lipoxygenase inhibitor
(B) The major adverse effect of aspirin is gastrointestinal bleeding
(C) Aspirin can reduce normal body temperature
(D) Aspirin is a competitive inhibitor of platelet cyclooxygenase

40. Each of the following conditions is a classic histologic characteristic of chronic inflammation EXCEPT

(A) infiltration by mononuclear leukocytes
(B) infiltration by polymorphonuclear leukocytes
(C) proliferation of fibroblasts
(D) fibrosis
(E) tissue destruction

41. A 22-year-old woman reports the gradual onset and relentless progression of severe pain in the lower left quadrant of her abdomen. A pelvic exam determined that there was marked tenderness both upon direct palpation and upon manipulation of the cervix. A greenish-yellow discharge from the cervical os was noted, but a direct gram-stain of the discharge revealed no potential etiologic agents. Despite this finding, she was started on antibiotic therapy. Twenty-four hours later, laboratory culture of the discharge yielded growth of oxidase-positive, gram-negative diplococci on Thayer–Martin medium. A diagnosis of gonococcal salpingitis was made. One week post-therapy, the patient's symptoms were relieved and laboratory culture of her cervix revealed no pathogenic organisms. What is the patient's future prognosis?

(A) The patient may not be cured and will require constant monitoring of her cervical flora for the next 6 months
(B) The patient may not be cured and is therefore encouraged to abstain from sexual encounters or observe safe-sex practices for the next 6 months
(C) The patient is cured and requires no further monitoring
(D) The patient is cured, but faces an increased risk of subsequent episodes of pelvic inflammatory disease, infertility, and ectopic pregnancy

42. Loop diuretics, such as furosemide, are very useful in the treatment of edema due to cardiac or hepatic failure. The intense diuresis may be associated with

(A) an increase in glomerular filtration
(B) metabolic acidosis
(C) hypercalcemia
(D) hypokalemia
(E) a decrease in renal blood flow

Questions 43 and 44

A 10-year-old boy with a history of episodic dyspnea associated with wheezing has the following spirometric tracings before and after inhalation of a bronchodilator.

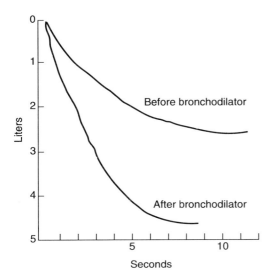

43. A possible pharmacotherapeutic approach to control this boy's symptoms may include

(A) antihistamines
(B) propranolol
(C) cromolyn sodium
(D) aspirin
(E) neostigmine

44. Inhalation of an irritant that stimulates the nonmyelinated "C fibers" beneath tight junctions between epithelial cells lining the airway lumen produces reflex bronchoconstriction via the

(A) intercostal nerves
(B) phrenic nerves
(C) vagus nerve
(D) hypoglossal nerve
(E) sympathetic nerve endings

45. Tay-Sachs is an autosomal recessive disease with an incidence of 1/3600 among the Ashkenazi Jewish population. Of the following values, which one is the frequency of the Tay-Sachs gene?

(A) 1/4
(B) 1/30
(C) 1/60
(D) 1/600

46. A 25-year-old sexually active woman is evaluated for her fourth acute urinary tract infection during the past 12 months. Her infections are characterized by frequency, urgency, dysuria, and *Escherichia coli* bacteriuria. Her recurrent infections are most likely due to

(A) overgrowth of highly resistant *E. coli* in her fecal reservoir
(B) passage of an infected renal calculus
(C) resistance of the bacteria to the drugs selected for treatment
(D) presence of a foreign body within the genitourinary tract
(E) colonization of the vaginal introitus with fecal Enterobacteriaceae

47. A healthy person is flying in an airplane that has been pressurized to 10,000 feet (523 mm Hg). Which of the following statements concerning the effects of this barometric pressure is true? It

(A) will not affect alveolar P_{O_2} because inspired oxygen remains at 0.21
(B) will be associated with significant desaturation of arterial hemoglobin
(C) will shift the subject's oxyhemoglobin dissociation curve to the left
(D) will decrease the vapor pressure of water in the airways
(E) will cause a modest reduction in arterial P_{O_2}

48. Dinitrochlorobenzene (DNCB) was applied to a patient's skin over a 1-cm² area on the right forearm. About 2 weeks later, a pruritic rash occurred at the site. It can be concluded that

(A) the patient lacks all T-cell–mediated immune function
(B) the patient suffers from DiGeorge syndrome
(C) the reaction would require an additional 2 weeks to develop on subsequent exposure to DNCB
(D) the reaction observed was most likely caused by CD4+ T cells

49. A diagnostic feature of rheumatoid arthritis is

(A) subcutaneous nodules that do not reveal urate crystals when biopsied
(B) swelling of distal interphalangeal joints
(C) asymmetrical or single joint involvement
(D) anti-immunoglobulin G
(E) anti-immunoglobulin E

Questions 50–54

A 53-year-old man with normal renal function was admitted to a local hospital with a 5-cm firm, right-neck tumor, proven on open biopsy to be metastatic squamous carcinoma. The patient received intravenous cisplatin together with mannitol. After 4 days, he reported 2 days of nausea and vomiting with concomitant decrease in urine volume. Fluids were encouraged, and 3 days later the patient was given bleomycin as a bolus. Two days after that, the patient was admitted to the hospital because of continued oliguria, nausea, vomiting, and generalized erythema of his skin. Laboratory tests indicated normal liver, but not kidney function. Chest roentgenogram showed diffuse pulmonary infiltrates, and rales could be heard from the chest.

50. Which one of the following statements most accurately describes why mannitol was included in the regimen? It

(A) decreases the nausea and vomiting associated with cisplatin
(B) reduces the transit time of cisplatin in the kidneys and decreases renal damage
(C) increases the metabolism of cisplatin and decreases its myelosuppression
(D) reduces plasma protein binding of cisplatin, allowing more free drug to enter tumors

51. Where was the renal toxicity most likely to occur?

(A) Glomeruli
(B) Proximal tubules
(C) Loop of Henle
(D) Distal tubules

52. What caused the pulmonary toxicity?

(A) A decrease in the metabolism of bleomycin
(B) A decrease in the excretion of bleomycin
(C) Activation of the immune response secondary to the presence of the tumor
(D) Loss of renal function

53. Which of the following mechanisms of action most accurately describes that of cisplatin?

(A) Covalent interactions with mRNA
(B) Covalent interactions with tRNA
(C) Blocking DNA transcription and replication
(D) Blocking dihydrofolate reductase
(E) Covalent interactions with rRNA

54. The antitumor mechanism of action of bleomycin involves all of the following factors EXCEPT

(A) inhibition of dihydrofolate reductase
(B) fragmentation of DNA
(C) interaction of the drug with Fe^{2+}
(D) interaction of the drug with O_2
(E) recognition of specific nucleotide sequences

55. A blood smear contains a cell with a prominent Barr body. This cell probably is

(A) an eosinophil
(B) a neutrophil
(C) a basophil
(D) a monocyte
(E) a lymphocyte

56. A 56-year-old woman with a history of ovarian cancer treated by chemotherapy several years ago presents to a clinic with complaints of fatigue and the recent development of small hemorrhages on her arms. She has the following lab values: Hb, 9.6 g/dl; WBC, 2900/μl; platelets, 56,000/ml. A bone marrow aspirate is hypercellular and contains approximately 10% blasts (normal < 5%) with megaloblastic morphologic changes in the red cell precursors and megakaryocytes with abnormal nuclei. Cytogenetic analysis reveals a clone with a deletion of the long arm of chromosome 7. What diagnosis best fits her condition?

(A) Preleukemia (myelodysplastic syndrome)
(B) Megaloblastic anemia
(C) Acute lymphocytic leukemia
(D) Acute nonlymphocytic (myeloid) leukemia
(E) Chronic myelogenous leukemia

57. A newly isolated virus has a genome consisting of seven pieces of single-stranded RNA. When polyribosomes from infected cells are isolated, they are found to be associated with RNA molecules and are complementary in sequence to the genomic RNA isolated from purified virus particles. Which one of the following statements about this virus is most likely to be true?

(A) At least seven different proteins are encoded by the virus
(B) Naked RNA extracted from virus particles is infectious if introduced directly into susceptible cells
(C) The virus genome is composed of positive-polarity RNA molecules
(D) The virion RNA is replicated by a cellular polymerase

58. Chlorpromazine is an aliphatic derivative of phenothiazine that is useful in the treatment of schizophrenia. Which of the following neurologic side effects is most likely to appear after months of therapy?

(A) Seizure-like activity
(B) Akathisia
(C) Parkinsonism
(D) Orthostatic hypotension
(E) Tardive dyskinesia

59. Rapid diagnosis and determining the species of the causative agent is essential for which of the following life-threatening infections?

(A) Malaria
(B) Chronic Chagas disease
(C) Amebic dysentery
(D) Mucocutaneous leishmaniasis
(E) Giardiasis

60. Dexamethasone is a corticosteroid that is useful in certain forms of hypersensitivity reactions or inflammation. Significant adverse effects limit the use of dexamethasone in either large doses or prolonged administration. Important considerations include

(A) the mineralocorticoid activity of dexamethasone
(B) direct stimulation of phospholipase A_2
(C) suppression of the response to infection or injury
(D) stimulation of endogenous adrenocorticotropic hormone
(E) hypoglycemia

61. All of the following statements concerning action potentials recorded simultaneously from slow and fast myocardial fibers (illustrated below) are correct EXCEPT

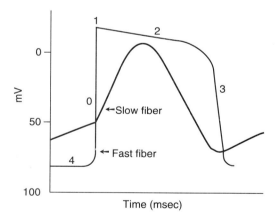

(A) the slow fiber was likely to be present in sinoatrial or atrioventricular nodes
(B) the fast fiber is typical of either atrial or ventricular myocardial cells
(C) in the fast fiber, phase 0 is due to opening of Na^+ channels
(D) in the fast fiber, phase 2 coincides with an increase in conductance to Ca^{2+}
(E) application of acetylcholine (ACh) increases the slope of phase 4 of the slow fiber

62. Each condition listed below is associated with an increased incidence of cryptorchidism EXCEPT

(A) short spermatic cord
(B) trisomy 21
(C) trisomy 13
(D) narrow inguinal canal
(E) deficiency of luteinizing hormone–releasing hormone

Questions 63–66

The following data were obtained from an arterial blood sample drawn from a hospitalized patient:

$$pH = 7.55$$
$$P_{CO_2} = 25 \text{ mm Hg}$$
$$[HCO_3^-] = 22.5 \text{ mEq/L}$$

Recall that $CO_2 = 0.03 \times P_{CO_2}$ (in mmol/L).

63. This patient's arterial blood findings are consistent with a diagnosis of

(A) metabolic alkalosis
(B) respiratory alkalosis
(C) metabolic acidosis
(D) respiratory acidosis

64. These findings indicate that the ratio of $[HCO_3^-]$ to dissolved CO_2 is

(A) 5:1
(B) 10:1
(C) 20:1
(D) 30:1

65. The data indicate that the CO_2 content is approximately

(A) 22 mmol/L
(B) 23 mmol/L
(C) 24 mmol/L
(D) 25 mmol/L
(E) 26 mmol/L

66. The major compensatory response for this patient's acid–base disorder is

(A) hyperventilation
(B) hypoventilation
(C) increased renal HCO_3^- excretion
(D) increased H^+ excretion

67. All of the following statements concerning insulin-dependent diabetes mellitus (type I) are correct EXCEPT

(A) sulfonylureas may be a useful adjuvant to insulin therapy
(B) use of recombinant "human" insulin has not eliminated problems of immunologic toxic effects
(C) insulin levels are routinely monitored
(D) ingestion of carbohydrates may be required to offset undesired hypoglycemia

Questions 68–70

A middle-aged man with a history of chronic cough with expectoration complains of shortness of breath and an increasing inability to exercise. A chest x-ray reveals cardiac enlargement, congested lung fields, and increased markings attributable to old infections. Spirometric tracings of a forced expiration after maximal inhalation are shown below for a normal subject (A) and the patient just described (B).

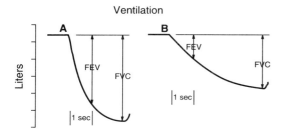

68. What conclusions can be drawn from the spirometric tracings of patient B?

(A) Total volume exhaled is near predicted
(B) Expiratory time is less than predicted
(C) The ratio of forced expiratory volume in 1 sec (FEV_1) to forced vital capacity (FVC) is near predicted
(D) The flow rate over most of the expiration is greatly reduced
(E) The elastic recoil of the lung is likely to be greater than predicted

69. A blood gas is drawn from patient B, and his arterial P_{CO_2} is 50 mm Hg (normal = 40 mm Hg). Which of the following factors is most likely to contribute to his CO_2 retention?

(A) An increased work of breathing
(B) An increased minute ventilation
(C) A large physiologic dead space
(D) A low physiologic shunt
(E) A rise in pH

70. A histopathologic hallmark of the disease in this patient is

(A) caseating necrosis
(B) noncaseating granuloma
(C) thickening of the interstitium of the alveolar wall
(D) plexiform arteriopathy
(E) hypertrophy of mucous glands

71. Zidovudine [(ZDV); formerly known as azidothymidine (AZT)] has all of the following properties EXCEPT

(A) ZDV reduces the chances of progression to AIDS in asymptomatic human immunodeficiency virus (HIV)-infected subjects
(B) ZDV improves the clinical symptoms of immunologic function, survival period, and quality of life of advanced AIDS patients
(C) ZDV is very toxic to bone marrow
(D) ZDV is effective only in the treatment of patients with advanced AIDS
(E) Prolonged treatment with ZDV (1–3 yrs) results in resistance to this drug

Questions 72 and 73

The figure below depicts log concentration–time curves for three drugs (X, Y, and Z) after identical amounts of each drug were administered as a bolus at time zero.

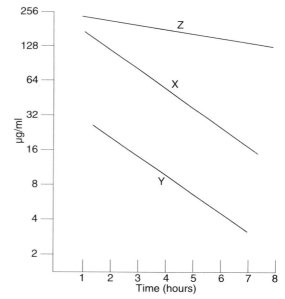

72. Which of the following statements regarding these drugs is correct?

(A) Volume of distribution (V_d) of X = Z < Y
(B) Half-time of elimination ($t_{1/2}$) of X = Y > Z
(C) Clearance of X (CL_X) = CL_Y
(D) CL_Z > CL_X
(E) Elimination rate constant (k) of X < (k) of Y

73. If drugs X, Y, and Z were independently infused in equal amounts at a constant rate, then based on the data from the figure above which of the following statements is most accurate?

(A) At steady state, [X] > [Z]
(B) At steady state, [X] = [Y]
(C) Z would require more time to reach a steady state than either X or Y
(D) X would reach a steady state faster than Y

74. For a patient trying to prevent intercourse-related recurrent urinary tract infections, which of the following antibiotics would be the most effective and economical when administered only once after coitus?

(A) Cephalexin
(B) Nitrofurantoin
(C) Trimethoprim-sulfamethoxazole
(D) Ciprofloxacin
(E) Penicillin G

75. In the lung, mean capillary pressure, negative interstitial fluid pressure, and interstitial fluid colloid osmotic pressure tend to move fluid out of the circulation. These forces are balanced by plasma colloid osmotic pressure. The Starling equilibrium for capillary exchange suggests that a slight amount of filtration at the capillaries occurs (usually offset by lymphatic drainage). If the permeability (reflection coefficient) of the lung remains constant, which of the following circumstances could lead to pulmonary interstitial edema?

(A) Increased left atrial pressure
(B) Decreased right atrial pressure
(C) Increased circulating albumin
(D) Sympathetic stimulation of lymphatic smooth muscle

76. A patient must be evaluated because of thrombocytopenia. The patient is a 55-year-old, previously well man, who was admitted to the hospital yesterday because of pneumonia. Antibiotic therapy was started, and his temperature continues to spike but is lower than on admission. On admission, his hemoglobin was reported to be 13 g/dl, white blood cell count was 9000/μl, and platelets 70,000/ml. The next laboratory study that should be done is

(A) bone marrow examination
(B) bleeding time
(C) examination of the peripheral smear
(D) platelet aggregation studies
(E) antiplatelet antibody detection tests

77. Type II (non–insulin-dependent) diabetes mellitus has several important clinical and pathologic features, including all of the following EXCEPT

(A) no human leukocyte antigen (HLA) association
(B) approximately 10% concordance in identical twins
(C) onset in the third or later decade of life
(D) no insulitis

78. A patient has hyperthyroidism, which is thought to have occurred due to elevated circulating levels of an immunoglobulin antibody (long-acting thyroid stimulator). Which one of the following statements can be made with accuracy?

(A) Injection of thyrotropin-releasing hormone (TRH) will result in a brisk increase in thyroid-stimulating hormone (TSH)
(B) The patient's circulating free thyroxine levels will be decreased
(C) There will likely be an overall decrease in the size of the patient's thyroid gland
(D) The patient will most likely have tachycardia

Questions 79 and 80

79. A 76-year-old man is admitted to the hospital with urinary retention as a consequence of benign prostatic hyperplasia. A catheterization performed in the emergency room drained 1500 ml of amber urine. The patient subsequently developed a significant postobstructive enuresis with a urine output of 100 to 150 ml/hr. The best explanation for this physiologic diuresis is

(A) excessive aldosterone secretion
(B) urea excess and volume overload
(C) decreased glomerular filtration rate (GFR)
(D) decreased tubular permeability
(E) increased renal blood flow

80. After 48 hours, the patient's excessive urine output is persisting, and he is not replacing his volume loss with oral fluid intake. The best explanation for this pathologic postobstructive diuresis is

(A) increased GFR
(B) urea excess and volume overload
(C) lack of tubular response to antidiuretic hormone and aldosterone
(D) decreased glomerular permeability
(E) increased renal blood flow

81. A tumor impinging upon the pterygopalatine fossa has the potential to affect all of the following structures EXCEPT the

(A) pterygopalatine ganglion
(B) maxillary division of CN V
(C) infraorbital artery
(D) pterygoid venous plexus

82. The modified Jones criteria are employed for the diagnosis of which of the following cardiac diseases?

(A) Secondary hypertension
(B) Secondary cardiomyopathy
(C) Acute rheumatic fever
(D) Cyanotic heart disease
(E) Syphilitic carditis

83. Hepatitis B vaccine should be offered to individuals significantly exposed to hepatitis B virus (HBV) infectious material when the exposed person's serum contains

(A) HBV surface antigen (HBsAg)
(B) hepatitis B e antigen (HBeAg)
(C) anti-HBc (core) antibodies
(D) anti-HBe antibodies
(E) no serologic markers of HBV infection

84. Human retroviruses have which one of the following characteristics? They

(A) do not fully transform cells in vitro and may lyse cells under certain conditions
(B) are exclusively lentiviruses
(C) exhibit B-type particle morphology
(D) resemble animal retroviruses in that they contain only *gag, pol,* and *env* genes

85. When histologically benign neoplasms prove fatal, they most likely do so because they

(A) cause extensive bleeding
(B) are multifocal
(C) fail to invoke an immune response
(D) interfere with organ function
(E) transform into carcinoma

86. Cancer of the breast that presents as a lump in the lower medial quadrant of the right mammary gland probably involves which one of the following lymph node groups?

(A) Internal thoracic nodes
(B) Supraclavicular nodes
(C) Anterior axillary nodes
(D) Deltopectoral nodes

87. In the general format of the Henderson-Hasselbalch equation:

$$\log\left(\frac{[\text{protonated form}]}{[\text{unprotonated form}]}\right) + pK'_a = pH$$

Phenobarbital is a weak acid. In an emergency situation, a useful maneuver to hasten its elimination in an intoxicated person might be

(A) inhalation of CO_2
(B) infusion of $NaHCO_3$
(C) infusion of NH_4Cl
(D) induction of P450 enzymes with a separate barbiturate
(E) infusion of dextrose

88. HLA typing of a disputed paternity case involving two children showed the following results:

Mother	A1, ?, B5, B7
Child 1	A1, A3, B5, B12
Child 2	A1, A9, B7, B17
Alleged father	A3, A9, B12, B17

Which of the following statements is correct?

(A) The alleged father is excluded as the true father of child 1
(B) Child 1 shares one HLA haplotype with child 2
(C) The alleged father is excluded as the true father of child 2
(D) The mother is homozygous for HLA–A1

89. Parkinsonism is a common neurologic movement disorder characterized by muscle rigidity, akinesia, flat facies, and tremor. Structural pathologies, especially in the basal ganglia and associated areas, are accompanied by an imbalance in dopaminergic and cholinergic activitites. Parkinsonism can be treated by all of the following modalities EXCEPT

(A) increasing the central nervous system (CNS) production of newly synthesized dopamine
(B) inhibition of monoamine oxidase (MAO) activity
(C) preventing the further loss of dopaminergic cells in the CNS
(D) prolonging the half-life of acetylcholine (ACh) at CNS synapses
(E) providing a centrally acting dopaminergic agonist

Questions 90 and 91

A 70-year-old woman is brought to the emergency room by her daughter, who noticed that her mother is not as energetic as she previously was. In the emergency room, the patient relates a history of increasing fatigability and shortness of breath over the past several months. On examination, the patient has elevated neck veins, rales in the back, and a third heart sound (S_3 gallop rhythm). Chest x-ray reveals an enlarged cardiac silhouette and increased vascular markings. The patient has a heart rate of 90 and a blood pressure of 150/100.

90. Based on the above history and physical examination, the patient is most likely to have

(A) atrial fibrillation
(B) ventricular paroxysmal tachycardia
(C) congestive heart failure
(D) adult respiratory distress syndrome
(E) rebound hypertensive crisis

91. A hypothetical series of pressure–volume loops of the left ventricle of a control subject and the above patient before and after digitalis is shown below. Based on these data, which one of the following groupings is correct?

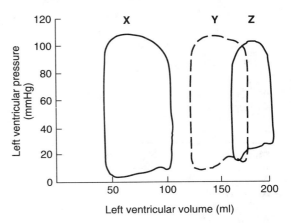

(A) X: control; Y: before digitalis; Z: after digitalis
(B) X: control; Z: before digitalis; Y: after digitalis
(C) Z: control; X: before digitalis; Y: after digitalis
(D) Z: control; Y:before digitalis; X: after digitalis

92. An analysis of chromosomal DNA, using the Southern blot technique, involves the following five major steps:

1. Autoradiography
2. Blotting
3. Cleavage
4. Electrophoresis
5. Hybridization

Which of the following sequences of steps best illustrates this technique?

(A) 1 2 3 4 5
(B) 1 3 2 4 5
(C) 3 5 2 4 1
(D) 3 2 5 4 1
(E) 3 4 2 5 1

93. Erythroblastosis fetalis is an example of which one of the following responses?

(A) Anaphylactic reactions (type I immunity)
(B) Cytotoxic reactions (type II immunity)
(C) Immune complex reactions (type III immunity)
(D) Cell-mediated immunity (type IV immunity)
(E) Arthus reaction

94. Lidocaine is the prototype of an amide local anesthetic and as such is

(A) free of potential central nervous system (CNS) side effects
(B) free of potential cardiac adverse effects
(C) rapidly metabolized by plasma cholinesterases
(D) a Na^+-channel blocker, especially in small, myelinated nerve fibers
(E) inappropriate for use in spinal anesthesia

95. During a thoracentesis, a needle is passed into the pleural cavity through the seventh intercostal space at the posterior midaxillary line. This thoracentesis pierces all of the following muscles EXCEPT the

(A) internal intercostal muscle
(B) serratus anterior muscle
(C) transverse thoracis muscle
(D) levator costarum muscle

96. The following data were obtained on a serum sample from a 3-year-old patient. G1m is an allotypic variation on IgG1.

Antibody	Serum	RBC coating	Hemagglutination
Anti-G1m(a)	none	Anti-G1m(a)	+
Anti-G1m(a)	Patient's	Anti-G1m(a)	−
Anti-G1m(f)	none	Anti-G1m(f)	+
Anti-G1m(f)	Patient's	Anti-G1m(f)	+
Anti-G1m(x)	none	Anti-G1m(x)	+
Anti-G1m(x)	Patient's	Anti-G1m(x)	−
Anti-G1m(z)	none	Anti-G1m(z)	+
Anti-G1m(z)	Patient's	Anti-G1m(z)	+

+ = agglutination.
− = no agglutination.

Which one of the following is the child's G1m type?

(A) ax
(B) fx
(C) zx
(D) z

97. In the figure below, volume–pressure curves from three subjects of the same age, sex, and body size are shown. If subject B is normal, which one of the following statements is most accurate?

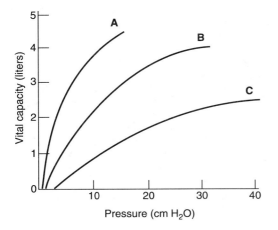

(A) Subject A has a stiff lung (fibrosis)
(B) Subject A has a flabby lung (emphysema)
(C) Subject A has a higher elastic recoil pressure than the other subjects
(D) Subject C is likely to have a higher functional residual capacity
(E) Subject C has the lowest elastic recoil pressure of the three

98. The Food and Drug Administration (FDA) has announced that it will test vaccines against HIV (the human immunodeficiency virus that causes AIDS) with the least potential for causing the disease and the best chance of inducing protective immunity. Which of the vaccination reagents listed is most likely to be tested?

(A) An attenuated virus that does not cause disease in monkeys
(B) A recombinant HIV DNA in a vaccinia virus to induce host cells to produce only the HIV p24 protein, and then antibodies to p24 protein
(C) A denatured, purified CD4 (T4) protein to cause the host to mount an immune response to the HIV-infected CD4+ cells
(D) A human monoclonal antibody that reacts with the intact CD4 (T4) receptor

99. An 86-year-old man has diminished vibratory sensation at the knees and toes, although his reflexes are intact, temperature sensation is normal, and he feels well apart from headaches. What is the most likely explanation?

(A) Peripheral neuropathy
(B) Normal age-related change
(C) Spinal cord lesion
(D) Small strokes
(E) Brain or brain stem tumor

100. Factors that distinguish cardiogenic pulmonary edema from noncardiogenic edema include which one of the following?

(A) Decreased pulmonary capillary pressure
(B) Decreased protein content of the edema fluid
(C) Slow resolution of edema with pharmacologic therapy
(D) Increased Na+ content of the edema fluid

101. Endorphins and enkephalins are the major chemical groups of the neuroactive opioids. Although they are distinct chemical and physiological peptides, endorphins and enkephalins are similar in that they share which one of the following characteristics? They are

(A) derived from a common precursor molecule, pro-opiomelanocortin
(B) synthesized primarily in the anterior pituitary of man
(C) found in the central nervous system even following hypophysectomy
(D) endogenous ligands for only one type of opioid receptor
(E) both primarily antinociceptive by suppressing substance P–containing nerve endings of the spinal cord

102. Ceftriaxone has replaced penicillin G as the drug of first choice for the treatment of gonorrhea because ceftriaxone

(A) is very effective when given orally
(B) is bactericidal by inhibiting protein synthesis in *Neisseria gonorrhoeae*
(C) is often effective in gonococci that synthesize β-lactamase
(D) does not cause a hypersensitivity reaction
(E) is less expensive than penicillin G (per dose)

103. True statements about the enzyme reverse transcriptase include which one of the following? It is

(A) commonly carried by those RNA viruses with a negative-polarity genome
(B) not found in retrovirus particles
(C) a viral oncogene product
(D) an enzyme possessing both DNA- and RNA-dependent polymerase activities
(E) commonly synthesized in normal eukaryotic cells

104. Cromolyn sodium is now the first-line agent for the treatment of mild to moderate asthma, especially asthma in chidren associated with allergenic causes. Although its mechanism of action is unclear, cromolyn sodium's widespread use is due to its

(A) bioavailability after oral administration
(B) direct bronchodilating effect, making it useful in acute emergencies
(C) prophylactic potential secondary to inhibition of the release of inflammatory mediators
(D) immediate effect to reduce bronchospasm
(E) antimuscarinic effects

105. Each of the following arteries arises from the axillary artery EXCEPT the

(A) subscapular artery
(B) posterior humeral circumflex artery
(C) dorsal scapular artery
(D) brachial artery
(E) supreme thoracic artery

106. The correct order of coronary artery involvement in atherosclerosis (from most to least frequent) is

(A) left circumflex coronary artery, right coronary artery, left anterior descending coronary artery
(B) left main stem coronary artery, left anterior descending coronary artery, left circumflex coronary artery
(C) right coronary artery, right main stem artery, left anterior descending coronary artery
(D) left anterior descending coronary artery, right coronary artery, left circumflex coronary artery
(E) right coronary artery, left anterior coronary artery, left main stem coronary artery

Questions 107 and 108

107. A patient has been hospitalized for 6 weeks due to a variety of complications beginning with a bowel obstruction. He has had several operative procedures, one of which necessitated a transfusion of 3 units of packed red blood cells. He has been unable to eat, and has been on broad-spectrum antibiotics almost continuously. His prothrombin time (PT) and partial thromboplastin time (PTT) have recently been noted to be prolonged. Quantitative fibrinogen, thrombin time, and platelet count are all normal, and the defect was corrected when the patient's plasma was mixed with an equal volume of normal plasma. The most likely cause of the coagulation abnormality is

(A) an acquired inhibitor
(B) dilution of coagulation factors secondary to transfusions
(C) vitamin K deficiency
(D) folate deficiency
(E) von Willebrand's disease

108. The patient is not actually bleeding. Which of the following therapeutic interventions should be suggested?

(A) Watch and wait
(B) Give fresh frozen plasma
(C) Give parenteral vitamin K
(D) Give cryoprecipitate
(E) Discontinue the antibiotics

109. The eclipse phase of the virus replication cycle has which one of the following characteristics? It

(A) is defined as that time period after which the first virus particles are assembled
(B) denotes the time between virus entry into the cell and the time virus particles appear extracellularly
(C) is that part of the replication cycle during which virus particles cannot be recovered from the infected cells
(D) is comparable to the metaphase portion of mitosis

110. The graph below illustrates the levels of gonadotropic and ovarian hormones during the normal female menstrual cycle. Luteinizing hormone (LH) peaks on day 0. Which of the following statements best describes the hormonal influences here?

LH (mU/ml)
60
40
20
FSH (mU/ml)
20
10
0
Prog (ng/ml)
10
5
0
E2 (pg/ml)
200
100
17α-OH Prog (ng/ml)
2
1
0
Days from LH peak: −14 −10 −5 0 +5 +10 +14

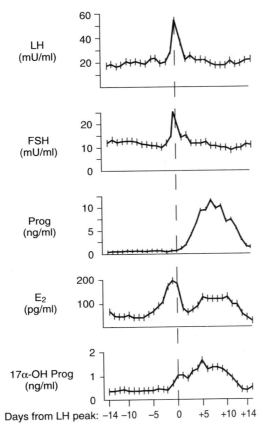

LH = luteinizing hormone
FSH = follicle-stimulating hormone
Prog = progesterone
E_2 = estradiol
17α-OH Prog = 17α-hydroxyprogesterone

(A) The dashed line indicates the onset of menstruation
(B) Ovulation occurs just prior to peak levels of plasma estradiol
(C) Progesterone levels are low to the left of the dashed line; therefore, the endometrium undergoes little structural change during this period
(D) Body temperature peaks to the left of the dashed line, under the influence of estradiol
(E) Elevated levels of follicle-stimulating hormone (FSH) and LH on day 0 cause theca-lutein and granulosa-lutein cells to secrete estradiol and progesterone

111. For the past 8 weeks, a scientist has developed rhinorrhea, conjunctival itching, a cough, and wheezing within 5 to 10 minutes of entering the animal facility where her experimental mice are housed. In the past week, she has begun to have wheezing and shortness of breath at night from 4 to 8 hours after working in the animal facility. Which of the following describes the late symptom complex? It is

(A) induced by mast cells triggered by rodent antigen with IgE
(B) a result of complement-mediated cytotoxicity
(C) not blocked by corticosteroids
(D) blocked by antihistamines

112. In the figure below, glucose transport — glucose that is filtered, excreted, and reabsorbed — is plotted against plasma concentrations. Which of the following statements about this figure is most accurate?

Glucose titration curve
Filtered
Excreted
Reabsorbed
Glucose transport (mg/min)
600
500
400
300
200
100
0
0 100 200 300 400 500 600 700 800
Plasma glucose concentration (mg/dl)

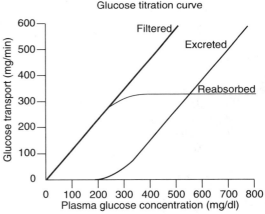

(A) The glomerular filtration rate (GFR) cannot be calculated from this figure
(B) Glucose appears in the urine even at normal glucose concentrations (100 mg/dl)
(C) Glucose is actively secreted into renal tubules at concentrations over 200 mg/dl
(D) At approximately 300 mg/dl, the tubular transport of glucose is saturated

113. Systemic lupus erythematosus (SLE) is characterized by immune system derangement and chronic inflammatory disease affecting multiple organ systems. Commonly observed features of SLE include all of the following EXCEPT

(A) anemia
(B) anti–double-stranded DNA antibodies
(C) anti-histone antibodies
(D) positive Venereal Disease Research Laboratory (VDRL) test
(E) overproduction of complement factors

114. Distention within the gastrointestinal tract produces contraction of the nearby proximal segment and relaxation in the close distal segment. This peristaltic reflex and movement towards the anus is primarily due to

(A) vagal input
(B) postganglionic sympathetic fibers
(C) afferent sensory nerve fibers
(D) central input
(E) the myenteric plexus

115. Gross and microscopic characteristics of Crohn's disease include all of the following EXCEPT

(A) a nonspecific transmural inflammation and fibrosis affecting all layers of gut serosa
(B) a flattening and fusion of surface villi in non-ulcerated mucosa
(C) fibrous structures that narrow the lumen of the ileum
(D) many recently developed lymphoid aggregates within the bowel wall
(E) inflammatory pseudopolyps

116. A common infection in American children that is characterized by pruritus ani is caused by

(A) *Necator americanus*
(B) *Ascaris lumbricoides*
(C) *Enterobius vermicularis*
(D) *Trichuris trichiuria*
(E) *Onchocerca volvulus*

117. When measuring the force developed during muscle contraction in which length remains constant (isometric contraction), force is

(A) directly proportional to initial length (preload) over a large range (1 cm to 3 cm)
(B) independent of the strength of electrical stimulation
(C) increased as a function of frequency of stimulation
(D) equal to afterload
(E) maximal when free intracellular Ca^{2+} is sequestered by the sarcoplasmic reticulum

118. An individual with a significant (20-mm) reaction to purified protein derivative (PPD) who has never had antitubercular drugs probably has

(A) miliary tuberculosis
(B) a calcified focal lesion visible on chest x-ray
(C) deficient cell-mediated immunity
(D) viable *Mycobacterium tuberculosis* in some body organ
(E) progressive chronic lung disease

119. Each statement below concerning the thyroid gland is true EXCEPT

(A) it is contained within a capsule
(B) iodide enters follicular cells by passive diffusion
(C) parafollicular cells synthesize calcitonin
(D) follicular cells secrete iodine
(E) iodination of thyroglobulin occurs at the apical border of the follicular cell

120. Each statement below concerning lipoproteins is true EXCEPT

(A) triglyceride from dietary fat is transported in chylomicrons
(B) very low-density lipoprotein (VLDL) is a precursor of both low-density lipoprotein (LDL) and high-density lipoprotein (HDL)
(C) the action of lipoprotein lipase on lipoproteins results in an increase in density
(D) the apoprotein components of plasma lipoproteins are synthesized in the liver and intestine
(E) apoprotein B of LDL is the recognition factor for binding to the LDL receptor

Questions 121–123

A 23-year-old woman traveled to Kenya. She was in good health and had been immunized against all of the major disease groups. While in Kenya, she took chloroquine and pyrimethamine–sulfadoxine prophylactically for malaria. After 2 months in Kenya, she developed a fever, abdominal pain, nonbloody diarrhea, severe back pain, and loss of mobility. Her diagnosis was schistosomiasis.

121. What drug is most likely to be used to treat the schistosomiasis?

(A) Metronidazole
(B) Quinacrine
(C) Suramin
(D) Praziquantel
(E) Niclosamide

122. The antimalarial chloroquine has all of the following actions EXCEPT

(A) intercalation with double-stranded DNA
(B) reduction of intracellular pH and cellular invasiveness of the parasite
(C) prevention of DNA replication
(D) inhibition of DNA transcription
(E) inhibition of folic acid synthesis

123. All of the following statements about schistosomes are true EXCEPT

(A) adult worms multiply in humans
(B) the male and female sexes are separate
(C) adult worms can migrate to the lungs of humans
(D) humans become infected after contact with contaminated water
(E) intense transient itching often follows infection

124. A human myeloma protein (IgM with kappa light chains; IgM, κ) is used to immunize a rabbit. The resulting antiserum is then absorbed with a large pool of IgM purified from normal human serum. Following this absorption, the rabbit antiserum is found to react only with the particular IgM myeloma protein used for immunization. With which of the following specific portions of the IgM, κ myeloma protein would this antiserum react?

(A) Constant region of the μ chain
(B) Constant region of the κ chain
(C) J chain
(D) Variable regions of the μ and κ chains

125. During portal hypertension, varices may form in each of the following sites EXCEPT the

(A) esophagus
(B) spleen
(C) terminal rectum
(D) abdominal wall
(E) jejunum

126. The incubation period for hepatitis B is

(A) less than 15 days
(B) 15 to 40 days
(C) 40 to 60 days
(D) 60 to 160 days
(E) more than 160 days

127. Women who are susceptible to recurrent urinary tract infections with Enterobacteriaceae differ from women who never have infections in that their

(A) vaginal secretions have a much higher pH
(B) vaginal epithelial cells demonstrate increased receptor sites (adherence) for *Escherichia coli*
(C) fecal reservoirs contain more virulent *E. coli*
(D) urethras are abnormally narrow
(E) bladder capacities are much smaller

Questions 128–130

A previously healthy 60-year-old man passed out while playing with his grandchildren. Although he quickly regained consciousness and became fully alert, his family called an ambulance. The emergency medical team found no abnormalities on the electrocardiogram or on physical examination. However, the patient was admitted to the coronary care unit of a local hospital. During the evening, the patient was noted to have a fast rhythm with a wide complex on his monitor followed by hypotension and loss of consciousness.

128. After electrical cardioversion with 200 watt seconds of direct current, possible therapy may include

(A) intravenous propranolol
(B) digitalis
(C) intravenous lidocaine
(D) intravenous diltiazem
(E) epinephrine

129. Blood is drawn from the patient serially over the next 8 to 48 hours, and serum enzyme studies are consistent with a diagnosis of myocardial infarction. The most likely change noted was

(A) a decrease in aspartate aminotransferase
(B) an elevation in creatine kinase–muscle brain isoenzyme (CK-MB)
(C) an increase in lactate dehydrogenase isoenzyme (muscle)
(D) a decrease in pseudocholinesterase

130. A radionuclide scan (with technetium-99m pyrophosphate) performed 48 hours after the initial incident in the hospital indicates significant damage to the anterior wall of the left ventricle. Subsequent coronary artery angiography most likely shows occlusion of the

(A) right coronary artery
(B) left circumflex artery
(C) coronary sinus
(D) left anterior descending coronary artery
(E) atrioventricular nodal artery

131. Which one of the following statements best describes chondroblasts?

(A) They are endosteal cells capable of secreting proteoglycan
(B) They are perichondrial cells capable of secreting type II collagen
(C) They are periosteal cells capable of secreting type I collagen
(D) They show little mitotic activity
(E) They are filled with rough endoplasmic reticulum but lack a Golgi apparatus

132. A major difference between heparin and warfarin derivatives (e.g., Coumadin) — two useful anticoagulants — is that heparin

(A) is useful in pregnant women because it does not cross the placenta
(B) affects clotting factors present in blood
(C) is effective after oral administration
(D) is primarily used in chronic therapy
(E) therapy can be reversed by administration of vitamin K

133. Lovastatin is a newly available lipid-lowering drug. It is currently first-line therapy for patients who are at risk for myocardial infarction secondary to hypercholesterolemia. Its major mechanism of action is believed to be

(A) inhibition of 3-hydroxy-3-methylglutaryl coenzyme A (HMG CoA)
(B) enhancement of the secretion of very low-density lipoproteins (VLDLs) from the liver
(C) the binding of bile acids in the intestine
(D) enhancement of the clearance of triglyceride-rich lipoproteins by lipoprotein lipase
(E) reduction of high-density lipoproteins (HDLs)

134. Which sequence below is the correct order of epidermal maturation?

(A) Stratum basale, stratum spinosum, stratum lucidum, stratum granulosum, stratum corneum
(B) Stratum basale, stratum spinosum, stratum granulosum, stratum lucidum, stratum corneum
(C) Stratum basale, stratum granulosum, stratum spinosum, stratum lucidum, stratum corneum
(D) Stratum basale, stratum lucidum, stratum spinosum, stratum granulosum, stratum corneum
(E) Stratum basale, stratum lucidum, stratum granulosum, stratum spinosum, stratum corneum

135. Which one of the following statements concerning the venous sinuses of the cranium is true?

(A) The great vein of Galen joins the superior sagittal sinus to form the straight sinus
(B) The confluence of sinuses is formed from the straight, occipital, and petrosal sinuses
(C) The transverse sinuses become the internal jugular vein at the petrous portion of the temporal bone
(D) The cavernous sinus drains into the superior and inferior petrosal sinuses

136. A 27-year-old woman, who had four injections of DPT vaccine as an infant and a booster at age 6, received a deep laceration while on a camping excursion. What is the preferred treatment method and rationale?

(A) Equine tetanus immune globulin, because it will passively immunize her
(B) Human tetanus immune globulin, because it will stimulate her anamnestic response
(C) An aminoglycoside because it will control the growth of *Clostridium tetani*
(D) Tetanus toxoid, because it will stimulate her anamnestic response

137. Bromocriptine is an ergot derivative that has significant dopaminergic effects. It may be used to

(A) inhibit galactorrhea and amenorrhea associated with hyperprolactinemia
(B) promote lactation after parturition
(C) relieve nausea from a variety of causes
(D) stimulate growth hormone release in patients with acromegaly
(E) stimulate prolactin synthesis in normal subjects

138. Each structure below is lined by stratified squamous epithelium EXCEPT the

(A) mouth
(B) esophagus
(C) vagina
(D) peritoneum
(E) anal canal

139. Which of the following conditions is most likely to occur following trauma to the testis?

(A) Hydrocele
(B) Varicocele
(C) Hematocele
(D) Spermatocele
(E) Chylocele

140. In renal clearance, the amount filtered ($P_x \cdot C_x$) equals the amount excreted ($U_x \cdot \dot{V}$), where P_x is plasma concentration, C_x is plasma clearance, U_x is urine concentration, and $\dot{V}$ is urine flow.

If renal blood flow is 500 ml/min, the glomerular filtration fraction is 0.25, P_x is 100 mg/100 ml, U_x is 125 mg/ml, and $\dot{V}$ is 1 ml/min, then substance x is

(A) albumin
(B) inulin
(C) *para*-aminohippuric acid (PAH)
(D) actively secreted
(E) totally reabsorbed

141. A patient with median nerve palsy will exhibit all of the following defects EXCEPT

(A) an inability to oppose the thumb
(B) a claw hand deformity
(C) thenar atrophy
(D) an inability to flex digits two and three

142. Each microscopic feature below is characteristic of Alzheimer's disease EXCEPT

(A) neurofibrillary tangles
(B) neuritic plaques
(C) amyloid angiopathy
(D) Lewy bodies
(E) granulovacuolar degeneration

143. A rabbit is immunized with bovine serum albumin to which 2,4-dinitrophenol has been conjugated (DNP-BSA). Immune serum from the rabbit is obtained and placed in the center well of an Ouchterlony plate, with antigens in the outer wells as shown below. All of the following statements are correct EXCEPT

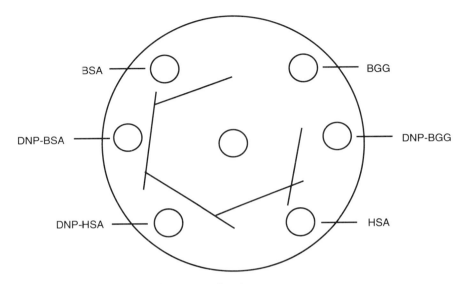

BSA = bovine serum albumin
HSA = human serum albumin
BGG = bovine gamma globulin
DNP-BSA = 2,4-dinitrophenol conjugated with BSA
DNP-HSA = 2,4-dinitrophenol conjugated with HSA
DNP-BGG = 2,4-dinitrophenol conjugated with BGG

(A) Both HSA and DNP-BGG are precipitated by the same antibodies so that there are overlapping spurs and no line of identity
(B) Anti-DNP antibodies react with DNP hapten on DNP-BGG, DNP-BSA, and DNP-HSA
(C) Some of the anti-BSA antibodies can cross-react with HSA, resulting in a line of partial identity
(D) None of the anti-BSA antibodies cross-react with BGG alone

144. Myeloid metaplasia with myelofibrosis is characterized by all of the following features EXCEPT

(A) hypocellular bone marrow
(B) normal levels of leukocyte alkaline phosphatase
(C) teardrop-shaped erythrocytes
(D) hepatomegaly
(E) splenomegaly

145. Serum samples from acute and convalescent blood of a patient were examined for their concentration of antiviral neutralizing (Nt) antibodies. Based on the antibody titer (i.e., concentration) data given below, what is the most likely cause of illness?

Serum	Coxsackievirus B1	Neutralizing antibody titers to Echovirus 4	Poliovirus type 1	HSV-1
Acute phase	256	256	64	128
Convalescent phase	512	2048	128	256

(A) Coxsackievirus B1
(B) Echovirus type 4
(C) Poliovirus type 1
(D) Herpes simplex virus type 1

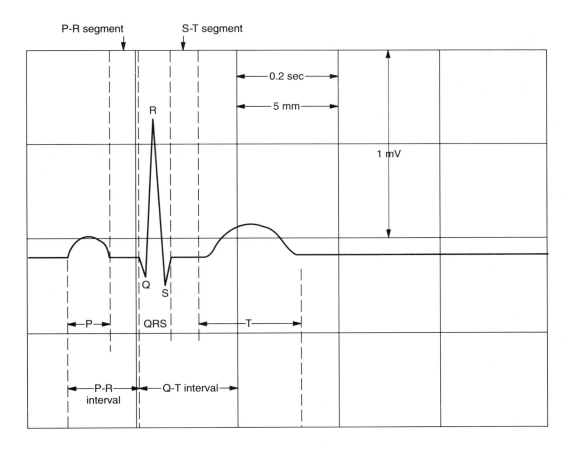

146. Each of the following statements concerning the normal electrocardiogram above is true EXCEPT
(A) the P-R interval is a measure of atrioventricular conduction
(B) the Q-T interval is a measure of duration of electrical systole
(C) the P loop is caused by atrial depolarization
(D) the T wave is caused by ventricular depolarization
(E) elevation in the S-T segment may be secondary to myocardial injury

147. In 1985, a couple (the father is blood type AB, Rh⁻, and the mother is B, Rh⁻) brought their 2-year-old child to the hematology laboratory for blood typing. The results of the hemagglutination assays are given below:

Serum	RBC	Results
None	Child's	−
Anti-A	Child's	−
Anti-B	Child's	+
Child's	A⁺	+
Child's	B⁺	−
Child's	Rh⁻, D⁺	−

+ = hemagglutination.
− = no hemagglutination.

Based on the assay results, which conclusion is valid?

(A) The child could not be the natural offspring of this couple
(B) The child is AB blood type
(C) The child's Rh type has not been definitively determined
(D) The child is not the offspring of the father

148. Each of the following statements concerning intercostal nerves is true EXCEPT that

(A) they are the anterior rami of the 12 thoracic spinal nerves
(B) they are connected to the sympathetic trunk by rami communicans
(C) the first intercostal nerve is joined to the brachial plexus
(D) they supply the anterior abdominal muscles
(E) they supply the parietal pleura

149. Despite the fact that a patient has always had B cells bearing antibodies that could react with ragweed antigen, he does not develop ragweed allergies until his second summer in a new city. Which one of the following reasons best explains why the patient developed a new allergy?

(A) He stopped producing T4⁺ helper cells that could provide help to ragweed-reactive B cells
(B) His T8 suppressor cells were turned into cytotoxic cells by exposure to ragweed antigen
(C) He lost the specific T8⁺ suppressor cells that held his B cells or their specific helpers in check
(D) His MHC class I genes mutated and now allow presentation of the antigen to the T4-helper population

150. Compared to skeletal muscle, most visceral (e.g., gut, reproductive) smooth muscle has which of the following properties? It

(A) is lacking in actin and myosin
(B) consumes more energy to sustain a given tension of contraction
(C) is made up of considerably larger fibers
(D) does not exhibit action potentials
(E) has far more voltage-gated Ca^{2+} channels and fewer Na^+ channels

151. Which one of the following coronary arteries probably is occluded when an infarct includes the area of the atrioventricular (AV) node?

(A) Left circumflex artery
(B) Left anterior descending artery
(C) Right coronary artery
(D) Marginal artery

152. If alveolar ventilation is doubled and CO_2 production is unchanged, then which one of the following will occur?

(A) Arterial P_{CO_2} (Pa_{CO_2}) will not change
(B) Alveolar P_{CO_2} (PA_{CO_2}) will double
(C) Arterial P_{CO_2} (Pa_{CO_2}) will decrease by half
(D) Alveolar P_{O_2} will double
(E) Alveolar P_{O_2} will not change

153. An important consideration in endocrine pharmacology is that many physiologic outcomes of hormone replacement therapy are dependent upon the rate at which exogenous hormones are administered. Continuous administration of high doses of gonadotropin-releasing hormone (Gn-RH) is most likely to

(A) stimulate release of follicle-stimulating hormone (FSH) but not luteinizing hormone (LH)
(B) stimulate relase of LH but not FSH
(C) restore normal ovulation in patients with hypothalamic disease
(D) block ovulation in normal subjects
(E) be useful in a patient with hypogonadotropic hypogonadism

154. Myasthenia gravis is an autoimmune disease typified by muscular weakness and increased fatigability, resulting from failure of neuromuscular transmission. Which one of the following drugs will exacerbate the symptoms of myasthenia gravis?

(A) Atropine
(B) Bethanechol
(C) Neostigmine
(D) Pralidoxime
(E) d-Tubocurarine

155. Pretreatment with the tricyclic antidepressant imipramine will decrease the antihypertensive effect of

(A) methyldopa
(B) clonidine
(C) propranolol
(D) captopril
(E) pargyline

156. Under which of the following circumstances will a graft-versus-host reaction occur? A and B represent different major histocompatability complex (MHC) haplotypes.

(A) Homozygous strain AA mouse spleen cells are injected into an irradiated strain AA neonate
(B) Strain AA x BB F_1 bone marrow cells are injected into an irradiated strain BB mouse, thymectomized as a neonate
(C) Strain AA skin cells are grafted to an irradiated strain BB mouse
(D) Strain BB spleen cells are injected into the F_1 progeny of AA and BB parents

157. A 19-year-old, recently married woman visits her family physician complaining of frequency and urgency of urination with burning pain in the vaginal area. Questioning of the patient does not reveal any recent history of systemic symptomatology; physical examination reveals a well-developed, well-nourished, healthy person. The presumptive diagnosis is uncomplicated urinary tract infection (UTI). The most probable etiologic agent is

(A) *Staphylococcus aureus*
(B) *Klebsiella pneumoniae*
(C) *Gardnerella vaginalis*
(D) *Escherichia coli*
(E) *Serratia marcescens*

Questions 158–161

Match each location of cellular function with the most appropriate structure.

(A) Golgi apparatus
(B) Endoplasmic reticulum
(C) Lysosome
(D) Mitochondrion
(E) Plasma membrane

158. Where many proteins are synthesized

159. Where growth factor receptors are primarily located

160. Where proteins are first glycosylated

161. Where sialic acid is added to proteins

162. The most common etiologic agents of bacterial endocarditis are

(A) staphylococci
(B) *Strongyloides stercoralis*
(C) *Necator americanus*
(D) anaerobic gram-positive cocci
(E) viridans streptococci

163. A young woman whose blood type is B, Rh^- receives blood from an A, Rh^+ donor after a car accident. The young woman has a subsequent transfusion reaction. Of the following reactions, which is most likely to occur?

(A) A subsequent fetus, who is B, Rh^+, might develop erythroblastosis fetalis
(B) The patient would have had no detectable antibodies against A or Rh antigens before the transfusion
(C) A subsequent fetus, who is Rh^-, is likely to develop erythroblastosis fetalis
(D) The transfusion reaction is related solely to naturally occurring antibodies against Rh antigen

164. Atropine, a prototype of a group of agents that acts like competitive antagonists at muscarinic receptors, has which of the following characteristics? It is

(A) restricted from entering the central nervous system (CNS) by the blood–brain barrier
(B) useful in treating postoperative urinary retention
(C) contraindicated in patients with bronchial asthma
(D) useful in increasing heart rate and reducing atrioventricular conduction time
(E) contraindicated for surgical procedures because it enhances bronchial secretions

165. If the pH and PO_2 remain constant, an increase in respiratory activity upon inhalation of CO_2 is likely to be primarily due to which of the following actions?

(A) Stimulation of J fibers in the lung
(B) Direct stimulation of nuclei in the dorsal region of the medullary center
(C) Conversion to H^+ in the cerebrospinal fluid (CSF) and subsequent stimulation of receptors in the ventral surface of the medulla
(D) Stimulation of carotid chemoreceptors

166. Combinations of anticancer drugs are often used for chemotherapy. An important underlying principle in selecting appropriate drugs for such combination therapy is that the drugs should

(A) have the same chemical structure
(B) stimulate each other's metabolism
(C) have similar mechanisms of antitumor activity
(D) have overlapping toxicities
(E) be substrates for similar resistance mechanisms

167. African trypanosomiasis (sleeping sickness) and malaria can be compared in which one of the following ways?

(A) Malaria and African trypanosomiasis are caused by different species of the genus *Trypanosoma*
(B) Both produce infections characterized by periodic febrile episodes
(C) The causative agents are obligate intracellular organisms
(D) Malaria is an insect-borne disease, while trypanosomiasis is a water-borne disease
(E) Erythrocytes are primary sites of parasitic development in the human host

168. Digitalis, the prototype of cardiac glycosides, is extensively used in congestive heart failure as well as several forms of cardiac dysrhythmias and has which of the following characteristics? It

(A) is positively inotropic and positively chronotropic
(B) increases intracellular Ca^{2+} by increasing the conductance for Ca^{2+} in voltage-sensitive channels
(C) has a high therapeutic index
(D) has a greater effect on cardiac rhythym during hypokalemia
(E) is vagolytic

169. Each of the following muscles helps dorsiflex the ankle EXCEPT the

(A) tibialis anterior
(B) peroneus tertius
(C) peroneus brevis
(D) extensor digitorum longus

170. All of the following statements concerning a healthy 3-year-old boy who develops hives after eating peanuts are correct EXCEPT

(A) complement activation is responsible for the development of the lesion
(B) histamine release occurs within the skin lesions
(C) the development of skin lesions is mediated by immunoglobulin E (IgE)
(D) aspirin administration is contraindicated
(E) mast cells release substances that mediate the hypersensitivity reaction

171. Propylthiouracil (PTU), which is useful in the treatment of some forms of hyperthyroidism, has which one of the following characteristics? It

(A) must be given parenterally
(B) does not cross the placenta or enter into breast milk
(C) immediately (within 24 hours) reverses many of the symptoms of Graves' disease
(D) is an inhibitor of both organification and peripheral deiodination of thyroxine
(E) is not used as a sole agent in the treatment of hyperthyroidism

172. Deposition of crystals of sodium urate, a purine metabolic by-product, causes the symptoms associated with intermittent attacks of gout. Agents that are useful in the palliative therapy of gout include all of the following EXCEPT

(A) acetaminophen
(B) acetylsalicylic acid (aspirin)
(C) allopurinol
(D) colchicine
(E) sulfinpyrazone

173. Which one of the following statements concerning oxidative phosphorylation is true?

(A) An agent that blocks a step in the electron transport chain will not inhibit oxidative phosphorylation
(B) The free energy stored in a proton gradient drives adensosine triphosphate (ATP) synthesis
(C) An uncoupler will inhibit oxygen consumption
(D) Inhibitors of ATP synthesis do not affect electron transport
(E) The P:O ratio of oxidized nicotinamide-adenine dinucleotide (NAD^+)-linked substrates is 2

174. Of the following viral categories, human immunodeficiency virus (HIV) is

(A) an endogenous retrovirus
(B) an example of an acute-transforming virus
(C) a replication-competent lentivirus
(D) an oncovirus

Questions 175–180

A mildly obese 20-year-old man presents to the emergency room at 5:00 A.M. He had ingested several six-packs of beer the evening before and had awakened at home with a sharp pain in his wrist at the radial–carpal articulation. The wrist is swollen and tender. The patient is slightly disoriented and ataxic but does not remember falling. X-rays of the wrist are negative. A slight fever is present.

175. The physician should order all of the following laboratory tests at this time EXCEPT

(A) synovial fluid analysis
(B) erythrocyte sedimentation rate
(C) C-reactive protein
(D) differential white blood cell count
(E) serum transaminase

176. Based on the information available, the most likely diagnosis is

(A) hyperuricemia
(B) Lesch-Nyhan syndrome
(C) osteoarthritis
(D) calcium hydroxyapatite deposition disease
(E) carpal tunnel syndrome

177. Synovial fluid analysis is done. The synovial fluid crystals are most likely composed of

(A) calcium oxalate
(B) calcium hydroxyapatite
(C) calcium carbonate
(D) sodium urate
(E) sodium oxalate

178. Biochemical studies confirm the suspected diagnosis. This patient suffers from lack of an enzyme whose product is

(A) 6-phosphogluconate
(B) citrulline
(C) inosinate
(D) oxaloacetate
(E) adenosine

179. The patient should be treated initially with

(A) adenosine replacement therapy
(B) azathioprine
(C) colchicine
(D) azidothymidine
(E) propoxyphene

180. For long-term therapy, the patient should be treated with

(A) acyclovir
(B) allopurinol
(C) amantadine
(D) acetazolamide
(E) ampicillin

181. Tetralogy of Fallot involves all of the following defects EXCEPT

(A) ventricular septal defect
(B) patent ductus arteriosus
(C) pulmonary valve stenosis
(D) dextroposed (overriding) aorta
(E) right ventricular hypertrophy

182. Each statement below concerning coenzymes is true EXCEPT

(A) their structure may contain nucleotides
(B) reduced nicotinamide-adenine dinucleotide (NADH) is a carrier of a hydride ion
(C) pyridoxal phosphate is a carrier of amino groups
(D) biotin becomes covalently bound to the enzyme
(E) thiamine is the precursor for the coenzyme that transports —CH_3 groups

183. Herpesviruses have which one of the following characteristics? They

(A) replicate exclusively in the cytoplasm of cells
(B) may remain latent in sensory ganglion neurons
(C) may lie dormant in epithelial cells of the skin between outbreaks of fever blisters
(D) cause recurring bouts of autoimmune disease

184. Each of the following statements concerning berry aneurysms is true EXCEPT that they

(A) are associated with chronic hypertension
(B) represent discontinuity of smooth muscle
(C) often are associated with adult polycystic kidney disease
(D) frequently are found at the bifurcation of cerebral arteries
(E) are not present at birth

185. Edema occurs in all of the following pathologic states EXCEPT

(A) cirrhosis of the liver
(B) congestive heart failure
(C) systemic hypertension
(D) kwashiorkor
(E) nephrotic syndrome

Questions 186 and 187

186. A 62-year-old man complains of urinary frequency, diminished force of his stream, inability to empty his bladder completely, and nocturia of four or five times. On rectal examination, the prostate is enlarged, smooth, symmetric, and nontender. The androgen most responsible for his prostate enlargement is

(A) testosterone
(B) dihydrotestosterone
(C) dehydroepiandrosterone
(D) androstenedione
(E) aldosterone

187. On further questioning, the patient reports frequent episodes of allergic rhinitis for which he takes large amounts of self-prescribed medication containing phenylpropanolamine. His symptoms of bladder neck outlet obstruction may be worsened by this drug because of its

(A) anticholinergic activity
(B) cholinergic activity
(C) sympathetic α-blocking properties
(D) sympathetic α-agonistic properties
(E) sympathetic β-agonistic properties

188. Nissl substance is a basophilic substance that is abundant in large motor neuron cells. Which of the following cellular components causes the basophilia of Nissl substance?

(A) DNA
(B) RNA
(C) Lipids
(D) Glycogen
(E) Synaptic vesicles

189. Paneth cells secrete which one of the following compounds?

(A) Lysozyme
(B) Pepsinogen
(C) Intrinsic factor
(D) Gastrin
(E) Hydrochloric acid

190. Which of the following types of necrosis most often follows a myocardial infarction?

(A) Coagulative
(B) Liquefactive
(C) Fat
(D) Caseous
(E) Gangrenous

191. The oxyntic (parietal) cells of the stomach secrete an electrolyte solution that contains a significant amount of HCl. Which of the following tends to inhibit this energy-requiring movement of H$^+$ into the gastric secretions?

(A) Histamine
(B) Acetylcholine
(C) Gastrin
(D) Food within the gut
(E) Acetazolamide

192. A 31-year-old man with hemophilia was found by serologic testing to have human immunodeficiency virus (HIV) infection. On routine chest x-ray, his right lung showed an infiltrate, which was proven to be caused by *Mycobacterium tuberculosis*. All of the following statements are true EXCEPT

(A) purified protein derivative (PPD) skin test might be nonreactive because of the immunodepression from HIV
(B) the virulence of *M. tuberculosis* makes it one of the early opportunistic infections in patients with HIV
(C) like *Mycobacterium avium-intracellulare, M. tuberculosis* is not transmitted from human to human, and treatment is not indicated
(D) within any mycobacterial population, there are drug-resistant mutants, making it necessary to use two or three antituberculous drugs whenever treating tuberculosis

193. A 6-year-old girl has been sick with life-threatening pyogenic infections since 3 months of age. Bacterial tests are positive for coagulase-positive staphylococci. Physical examination shows hepatosplenomegaly and general lymphadenopathies. A draining suppurative lymph node is on the left side of the neck. Immunoglobulin levels are: IgG, 1800 mg/dl; IgA, 200 mg/dl; IgM, 250 mg/dl. Of the following tests, which would be expected to give the most useful information?

(A) Basophil count
(B) CD4/CD8 T-cell ratios
(C) Assay of antibodies to tetanus and diphtheria toxoids within 1 week of the DPT booster
(D) Assay for the myeloperoxidase activity of neutrophils

Questions 194–204

Military operations in the Middle East have always been hampered by the effects of infectious disease. Those most frequently encountered are various diarrheas, hepatitis, sandfly fever, cutaneous leishmaniasis, and schistosomiasis; typhoid fever, malaria, and Congo–Crimean hemorrhagic fever have also been reported.

Sergeant Able reported to sick bay complaining of uncontrolled diarrhea, with six incidents during the past 24 hours. He was uncomfortable and tired but otherwise seemed to be improving. Upon examination, there were no remarkable findings. His temperature was normal. Examination of a stool specimen showed neither blood, leukocytes, nor highly motile bacteria.

194. What is the best form of treatment for Sergeant Able? He should

(A) be treated aggressively with intravenous rehydration and penicillin
(B) be treated by oral rehydration and loperamide
(C) be treated with metronidazole
(D) be sent back to his unit without treatment

195. How did Sergeant Able most likely acquire his infection? From

(A) a mosquito
(B) food bought at an outdoor market
(C) crackers in his ready-to-eat meal (REM)
(D) an alcoholic drink distilled in his barracks
(E) hot tea shared with Saudi soldiers

196. The organism most likely responsible for Sergeant Able's diarrhea is

(A) *Shigella dysenteriae*
(B) *Campylobacter jejuni*
(C) *Escherichia coli*
(D) *Plasmodium falciparum*
(E) *Entamoeba histolytica*

Sergeant Baker accompanied Sergeant Able to sick bay. Sergeant Baker's illness began violently 2 days ago, with spiking fever (40° C), pain, malaise, and massive diarrhea. Subsequently, he had up to 30 small, bloody, mucoid stools per day, with painful cramping and tenesmus, but little or no fever. Microscopic examination revealed leukocytes and blood in the stool. Although weak and uncomfortable, Sergeant Baker was not completely incapacitated.

197. Sergeant Baker is probably suffering from

(A) shigellosis
(B) cholera
(C) typhoid fever
(D) food poisoning
(E) amebiasis

198. What is the best form of treatment for Sergeant Baker?

(A) Oral rehydration only
(B) Intravenous rehydration only
(C) Oral rehydration and loperamide
(D) Oral rehydration and an appropriate antibiotic
(E) Blood transfusion and an appropriate antibiotic

An Iraqi officer, Colonel Kouyoumijian, was escorted to the hospital by Saudi military police. Colonel Kouyoumijian had no fever nor abdominal pain, but he seemed severely dehydrated and very weak. He related that he had left his bunker 3 days previously and had been living precariously, eating scraps and drinking from the river. Twelve hours previously, he had massive diarrhea, which continued almost unremittingly. A stool sample collected in the hospital upon admission was colorless and translucent. Microscopic examination showed no leukocytes nor blood, but numerous highly motile bacteria were present.

199. What is Colonel Kouyoumijian's most likely diagnosis?

(A) Amebic dysentery
(B) Viral enteritis
(C) Cholera
(D) Salmonellosis
(E) Shigellosis

200. Treatment should consist of

(A) ampicillin plus loperamide
(B) streptomycin plus oral rehydration
(C) tetracycline plus intravenous rehydration
(D) hyperimmune globulin plus loperamide
(E) kaopectate plus tetracycline

201. How should the organism responsible for Colonel Kouyoumijian's disease be cultured?

(A) Anaerobically
(B) In an alkaline medium
(C) In minimal glucose

Lieutenant Doug arrived at the hospital feeling very ill and confused. His temperature was 41° C, his liver and spleen were enlarged, and his abdomen was diffusely tender. A history, obtained with difficulty due to the patient's confused mental status, revealed that 5 weeks previously he had a fever of 40° C accompanied by a shaking chill, headache, muscle and abdominal pains, and a sore throat. At the time, he thought he had an attack of influenza. He got better without treatment, but, 3 weeks later, he again had chills, fever (40° C), and one bout of diarrhea. Again, he recovered without treatment, but after about 10 days, he felt ill enough to seek assistance.

202. Lieutenant Doug is most likely suffering from
(A) amebic dysentery
(B) Lyme disease
(C) typhoid fever
(D) food poisoning
(E) cat-scratch disease

203. The organism responsible for the condition described is in the genus
(A) *Salmonella*
(B) *Klebsiella*
(C) *Plasmodium*
(D) *Treponema*
(E) *Shigella*

204. Lieutenant Doug probably acquired the infection from
(A) a ready-to-eat meal (REM)
(B) Turkish coffee
(C) drinking water
(D) heterosexual intercourse

205. Chronic Chagas disease should be considered in patients from Central and South America presenting with which of the following signs and symptoms?
(A) Periodic fever and chills
(B) Cardiac conduction defects
(C) Multiple mucocutaneous lesions
(D) Persistent diarrhea
(E) Pneumonia

Directions: Each group of items in this section consists of lettered options followed by a set of numbered items. For each item, select the **one** lettered option that is most closely associated with it. Each lettered option may be selected once, more than once, or not at all.

Questions 206–210

For each vitamin listed below, select the metabolic process with which it is most likely to be associated.

(A) Synthesis of amino acids
(B) Synthesis of DNA
(C) Calcium metabolism
(D) Electron transport
(E) Pentose phosphate pathway

206. Pyridoxal phosphate (vitamin B_6)

207. Folic acid (pteroylglutamic acid)

208. Cholecalciferol (vitamin D_3)

209. Niacin (nicotinic acid)

210. Thiamine (vitamin B_1)

Questions 211–214

Match each structure listed below with the most appropriate opening in the diaphragm.

(A) Aortic hiatus
(B) Esophageal opening
(C) Vena caval foramen
(D) None of the above

211. Right phrenic nerve

212. Superior epigastric artery

213. Thoracic duct

214. Greater splanchnic nerve

Questions 215–218

Match each of the following descriptions with the appropriate lettered component in this micrograph of the trachea.

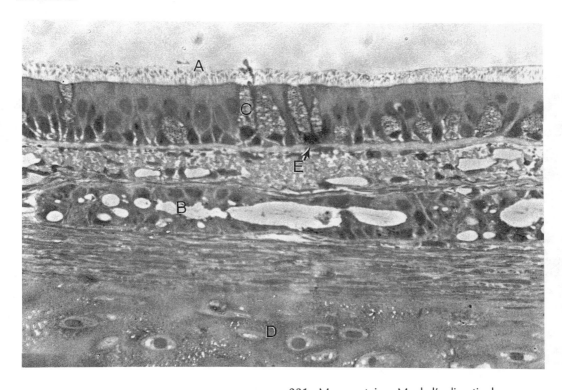

215. Basement membrane for the epithelium

216. Multicellular gland

217. Cell that secretes mucus

218. Flexible piece of avascular connective tissue that helps to maintain the tracheal lumen

Questions 219–222

Match each of the following descriptions with the appropriate segment or segments of the small intestine.

(A) Jejunum
(B) Ileum
(C) Both
(D) Neither

219. Contains well-developed plicae circulares

220. Contains many arterial arcades

221. May contain a Meckel's diverticulum

222. Has appendices epiploicae on its external surface

Questions 223–226

Match each description of developmental fate below with the appropriate portion of the early human blastocyst pre-embryo.

(A) Embryoblast
(B) Trophoblast
(C) Both
(D) Neither

223. Forms the cytotrophoblast and syncytiotrophoblast

224. Forms the epiblast and hypoblast

225. Derived from the zygote

226. Forms the placenta and chorion

Questions 227–230

For each abnormal process listed below, select the skeletal disease in which it is most likely to manifest.

(A) Osteogenesis imperfecta
(B) Osteopetrosis
(C) Achondroplasia
(D) Hereditary exostoses
(E) Osteoporosis

227. Sclerosis of cortical bone and narrowing of the medullary cavity

228. Osteochondromatosis that results in misdirected epiphyseal bone growth

229. Loss of cartilaginous spicules at the epiphyseal osteochondral junctions and premature ossification of these junctions

230. Thin, poorly formed bones that result in multiple fractures

Questions 231–236

For each skin condition listed below, select the type of vesicle that is most characteristic of that condition.

(A) Subcorneal
(B) Intraepithelial
(C) Subepidermal

231. Eczema

232. Pemphigus vulgaris

233. Pemphigoid

234. Dermatitis herpetiformis

235. Darier's disease

236. Miliaria

Questions 237–241

Match each description below with the appropriate lettered organ in the diagram.

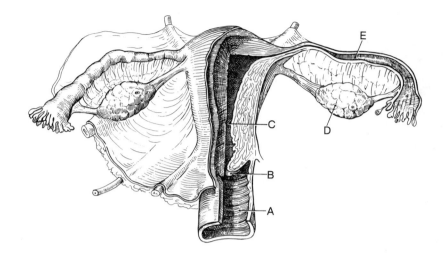

237. An organ covered by a simple cuboidal epithelium; its cortex contains stromal fibroblasts and gametogenic cells

238. An organ lined by a stratified squamous unkeratinized epithelium; it lacks glands

239. An organ with a zone of epithelial transition from simple columnar epithelium to stratified squamous unkeratinized epithelium

240. An organ with a simple columnar epithelium containing many ciliated cells and a few mucous-secreting cells

241. An organ with a simple columnar epithelium containing many mucus-secreting cells and a few ciliated cells; its glands become longer during the follicular phase of the menstrual cycle

Questions 242–245

Match each description below with the most appropriate sensory receptor.

(A) Pacini's corpuscles
(B) Ruffini's endings
(C) Meissner's corpuscles
(D) Merkel's cells
(E) Krause's end bulbs

242. Associated with free nerve endings; found in the stratum basale

243. Encapsulated receptor in the dermal papilla of thick skin; responsible for fine touch

244. Respond to pressure, vibration, and touch; consist of concentrically laminated, flattened cells

245. Terminal branches of an afferent nerve fiber; surrounded by a thin connective tissue capsule; found in the dermis and the joints

Questions 246–250

For each of the muscles listed below, select the nerve that is responsible for its innervation.

(A) Ansa cervicalis
(B) Facial nerve
(C) Greater auricular nerve
(D) Lesser occipital nerve
(E) None of the above

246. Sternomastoid muscle

247. Platysma muscle

248. Occipitofrontalis muscle

249. Omohyoid muscle

250. Geniohyoid muscle

ANSWER KEY

1-C	31-D	61-E	91-B	121-D
2-D	32-A	62-B	92-E	122-E
3-C	33-E	63-B	93-B	123-A
4-D	34-D	64-D	94-D	124-D
5-B	35-A	65-B	95-D	125-E
6-C	36-A	66-C	96-A	126-D
7-E	37-E	67-A	97-B	127-B
8-A	38-D	68-D	98-D	128-C
9-B	39-B	69-A	99-B	129-B
10-E	40-B	70-E	100-B	130-D
11-D	41-D	71-D	101-C	131-B
12-B	42-D	72-A	102-C	132-B
13-C	43-C	73-C	103-D	133-A
14-D	44-C	74-E	104-C	134-B
15-B	45-B	75-A	105-C	135-D
16-C	46-E	76-C	106-D	136-D
17-D	47-E	77-B	107-C	137-A
18-C	48-D	78-D	108-C	138-D
19-C	49-A	79-B	109-C	139-C
20-A	50-B	80-C	110-E	140-B
21-A	51-B	81-D	111-A	141-B
22-C	52-B	82-C	112-D	142-D
23-C	53-C	83-E	113-E	143-A
24-B	54-A	84-A	114-E	144-D
25-C	55-B	85-D	115-E	145-B
26-B	56-A	86-A	116-C	146-D
27-B	57-A	87-B	117-C	147-C
28-C	58-E	88-D	118-D	148-A
29-C	59-A	89-D	119-E	149-C
30-B	60-C	90-C	120-B	150-E

151-C	171-D	191-E	211-C	231-B
152-C	172-A	192-C	212-D	232-B
153-D	173-C	193-D	213-A	233-C
154-E	174-C	194-B	214-D	234-C
155-A	175-E	195-B	215-E	235-B
156-D	176-A	196-C	216-B	236-A
157-D	177-D	197-A	217-C	237-D
158-B	178-C	198-D	218-D	238-A
159-E	179-C	199-C	219-A	239-B
160-B	180-B	200-C	220-B	240-E
161-A	181-B	201-B	221-B	241-C
162-E	182-E	202-C	222-D	242-D
163-A	183-B	203-A	223-B	243-C
164-D	184-A	204-C	224-A	244-A
165-C	185-C	205-B	225-C	245-B
166-D	186-B	206-A	226-B	246-E
167-B	187-D	207-B	227-B	247-B
168-D	188-B	208-C	228-D	248-B
169-C	189-A	209-D	229-C	249-A
170-A	190-A	210-E	230-A	250-A

ANSWERS AND EXPLANATIONS

1. The answer is C. *(Log–dose response relationships)* Curves A, C, and D all reach about the same maximal response and, thus, are similar in efficacy. However, curve A is more potent than C, which, in turn, is more potent than D. Potency is based on the relative positions of the curves along the X axis. A competitive inhibitor would shift the curve to the right. For instance, curves A and C might be responses to an agonist in the absence (curve A) and presence (curve C) of a competitive inhibitor. Noncompetitive inhibitors decrease the efficacy (like a partial agonist might do). Thus, curves A and B might be the response to an agent in the absence (curve A) and the presence (curve B) of a noncompetitive inhibitor.

2. The answer is D. *(Biologic effects of androgens)* Although testosterone is required for normal spermatogenesis, it is involved in an important feedback inhibition pathway. Accordingly, introduction of high concentrations of testosterone can inhibit gonadotropin-releasing hormone production in the hypothalamus and interfere with important steps in spermatogenesis induced by leutenizing hormone (LH). In addition, testosterone can be metabolized to estrogens in men as well as women, and this estrogen formation can add to the inhibition of normal spermatogenesis. This effect is usually reversible in most mature men but can persist in a subset of anabolic steroid abusers. Testosterone is very likely to produce its well-known masculinizing effects in mature women and can produce feminization in men. Although testosterone has a significant myotrophic effect on muscle mass in children, it is never used in this age group because it causes closure of the epiphyses of long bones.

3. The answer is C. *(Anatomy of the spinal cord)* Access to the intrathecal space in mature subjects is most safely obtained via the lumbar spine, which is at L3–L4 inferior to the cessation of the spinal column (L1–L2). Although in some pediatric patients, access may be gained via the sacral region, in the adult, this is calcified and much more difficult to access. There is possibility of nerve damage to the cervical and thoracic spine secondary to trauma by the needle. An anterior approach at the level of the stellate ganglion (C6) presents the risk of damage to major vessels and nerve plexus.

4. The answer is D. *(Alveolar ventilation)* Alveolar ventilation is the product of respiratory rate × (tidal volume − dead space). In this situation total dead space (400 ml) is the sum of the patient's anatomic dead space (150 ml) and the ventilator's dead space (250 ml). Thus, if the total output of the ventilator is adjusted to 600 ml, then 200 ml of the alveolar volume will be delivered 20 times per minute and total minute alveolar ventilation will be 4 L/min.

5. The answer is B. *(Blood pressure regulation)* Angiotensin-converting enzyme (ACE) hydrolyzes the decapeptide angiotensin I to the vasoconstrictor octapeptide angiotensin II. Inhibition of this enzyme by a number of competitive antagonists is a new and useful way to lower blood pressure in some individuals. In addition to reducing circulating levels of the endogenous angiotensin II peptide, inhibition of ACE may have central effects, including a decrease in the dipsogenics effect of angiotensin II. Furthermore, angiotensin II appears to facilitate neurotransmission in the central and peripheral sympathetic nervous systems. Although angiotensin II is a potent stimulator of aldosterone secretion in the zona glomerulosa of the adrenal cortex, and inhibition of this effect might be expected to reduce blood pressure (by enhancing Na^+ excretion by the kidneys), there usually is little change in aldosterone levels because other endogenous secretagogues, including steroids, K^+, and minimal levels of angiotensin II, can maintain aldosterone secretion. Nonetheless, there is little indication to believe that the aldosterone level would actually increase, and if it did, this would result in Na^+ reabsorption, water retention, and an increase in arterial blood pressure.

6–8. The answers are: 6-C, 7-E, 8-A. *(Medical ethics)* If the physician's sole concern is not to harm the patient with unnecessary worry, the guiding principle is nonmaleficence. If her sole concern is to be able to benefit the patient with urography (which is impossible if the patient refuses because of concerns about the risks), the guiding principle is beneficence. Both are possible. Justice is irrelevant, and gratitude (e.g., for the patient's patronage) is at most marginally relevant.

If the physician decides to do whatever others of her profession do in like circumstances, she is acting without appeal to the independent ethical principles of beneficence and nonmaleficence. Depending on what the professional practice standard dictates, the disclosure decision might prove to be respectful of autonomy or strongly paternalistic, but the decision would still be guided by professional practice. Weak paternalism is entirely irrelevant because the patient is competent.

If the physician is guided by respect for the patient's preferences, she is acting with respect for her patient's autonomy. If the patient would want disclosure, it is possible that such disclosure could fail to benefit him or could even harm him, so neither beneficence nor maleficence is guiding the physician's thinking. Clearly, the basis for her thinking is independent of the usual practice of her profession.

9. The answer is B. *(Organophosphate exposure and inhibition of acetylcholinesterase)* Organophosphates are highly toxic insecticides that occasionally affect agricultural workers. They are also frequently the primary agent in chemical weapons. They are highly lipid-soluble and are absorbed through virtually all body parts, including the skin. They produce a cholinergic crisis secondary to inhibition of acetylcholinesterase, which involves nicotinic and muscarinic receptors, both centrally and systemically. Atropine decreases some of the muscarinic effects, including the bronchospasm and increased secretions of the airways. Mechanical ventilation may still be required if respiratory muscles are paralyzed. Pralidoxime, if given early enough, will help regenerate new cholinesterase and ultimately hasten reversal of the overdose.

10–13. The answers are: 10-E, 11-D, 12-B, 13-C. *(Whipple's disease)* The presenting symptoms are suggestive of an intestinal absorption disorder. Of the laboratory tests listed in the question, xylose absorption, small bowel x-rays, oral [^{14}C]triolein, and serum gastrin levels may be helpful for differential diagnosis.
Arthralgia, dilated lacteals, low-grade fever, and lymphadenopathy all suggest Whipple's disease. The diagnosis is established by the presence of macrophages positive for periodic acid–Schiff reagent. A normal serum gastrin level rules out Zollinger-Ellison syndrome. The treatment of choice is long-term antibiotic therapy. Whipple's disease should be treated with antibiotics, such as trimethoprim-sulfamethoxazole, for at least 1 year. Many intestinal absorption disorders, including Whipple's disease and Zollinger-Ellison syndrome, are characterized by anemia due to malabsorption of vitamin B_{12}. Supplementation with cyanocobalamin (vitamin B_{12}) should help to correct the patient's anemia.

14. The answer is D. *(Anatomy of the thorax)* Thoracic outlet syndrome describes compression of the lower trunk of the brachial plexus and the subclavian artery by an anomalous thirteenth (cervical) rib. Sensory changes occur over the distribution of the ulnar nerve; the phrenic nerves are not involved.

15. The answer is B. *(Coagulation and platelet function)* A significantly prolonged bleeding time deserves investigation before subjecting an individual to a surgical procedure, and the appropriate next step is platelet aggregation studies. Many of the inherited platelet function abnormalities result in serious bleeding, which can be life-threatening in a surgical setting. Defining the disease is obviously critical before making a therapeutic plan, which may carry its own risks. DDAVP is useful for controlling esophageal bleeding but is not routinely used in platelet dysfunction.

16. The answer is C. *(Varicella–zoster virus)* The lesions outside the dermatomal distribution are explained by depressed cell-mediated immunity. When varicella–zoster virus (VZV) goes outside a dermatomal distribution, it is because the affected person is immunosuppressed either from old age (> 65 years) or medication (in this case, chemotherapy). Thymidine kinase–negative mutants rarely occur, except in human immunodeficiency virus (HIV) patients on prolonged prophylaxis with acyclovir. Initial exposure to the infection always leads to viral latency in the dorsal ganglia.

17. The answer is D. *(Pathology of Barrett's esophagus)* Barrett's esophagus is a result of protracted reflux, due to lower esophageal sphincter incompetence, with the attendant increased exposure to acid, pepsin, and bile acids. Esophageal inflammation and ulceration occur followed by re-epithelialization and ingrowth of immature pluripotent stem cells. Rather than squamous epithelium, the new epithelium is columnar-lined with gastric or duodenal intestinal-type cells, which better tolerate prolonged acid exposure. Inflammation would only be absent in the case of postmortem ulceration and autolysis; such changes may be accompanied by "leopard spotting" — brown–black esophageal spots that form from acid digestion of hemoglobin.

18. The answer is C. *(Mechanism of action of viral envelopes)* Viral envelopes contain lipid bilayers (i.e., neutral lipids, phospholipids, and glycolipids) in addition to virus-specific proteins (i.e., glycoproteins and matrix proteins). It is the viral proteins on the envelope that bind to discrete cell receptors and recognize susceptible cells.

19. The answer is C. *(Toxicities of neoplastic agents)* Antineoplastic agents are associated with multiple and profound adverse effects. Some of these effects have particular significance for a small group of agents. Specifically, cisplatin is an unusual inorganic compound whose mechanism of action remains obscure. However, it is clear that it is initially concentrated in the kidneys where DNA intrastrand cross-linking of normal epithelium may occur. Hydration and diuresis are often required to counteract this adverse effect. Methotrexate inhibits DNA synthesis, and accordingly, its toxic effects are primarily depression of bone marrow and gastrointestinal epithelium. Bleomycin is a metal-chelating glycopeptide antibiotic that has a peculiar, and poorly understood, life-threatening side effect — pulmonary fibrosis. Busulfan is an alkylsulfonate alkylating agent that affects bone marrow function and also may cause pulmonary fibrosis, adrenal insufficiency, and increased skin pigmentation. Vincristine is a plant (*Vinca*) alkaloid that interacts with tubulin and is an important component of multidrug regimens for lymphomas and other cancers. It has a particularly significant neurotoxicity (areflexia and peripheral neuritis).

20. The answer is A. *(Anatomy of the female reproductive system)* Blood flows to the fallopian tubes through branches of the uterine vessels carried in the surrounding mesentery, which is called the mesosalpinx. The ovarian veins drain blood from the ovaries. The right ovarian vein drains into the inferior vena cava; the left ovarian vein drains into the left renal vein. Lymph from the cervix eventually drains into the internal and external iliac and obturator nodes. Visceral afferent nerves from the uterus follow two pathways: Fibers from the cervix follow the splanchnic nerves (nervi erigentes); however, the body of the uterus and uterine tubes send fibers in parallel to the sympathetic nerves.

21. The answer is A. *(Hypernatremia)* An increase in osmolality, especially due to increased plasma Na^+, excites osmoreceptors in the supraoptic nuclei of the hypothalamus. These nuclei release antidiuretic hormone that acts on distal renal tubular epithelium to conserve water while excreting Na^+. A decrease in plasma Na^+ has significant effects on other important hormonal and feedback systems for volume and osmolar regulation, including stimulation of aldosterone release and increased renin release from juxtaglomerular cells of the kidney.

22 and 23. The answers are: 22-C, 23-C. *(Medical genetics and cystic fibrosis)* The frequency of the cystic fibrosis (CF) gene is 1/40, the square root of the incidence of CF. Remembering the Hardy-Weinberg law, the gene frequency is equal to the square root of the incidence (q^2). If the incidence = q^2 = 1/1600, then the square root of the incidence, the gene frequency (q), = 1/40.

The proportion of normal siblings of CF individuals that would be expected to be carriers is 2/3. The recessive pattern of inheritance of CF sets each pregnancy at risk for the disease with a chance of one in four. This leaves a chance of two of the three individuals being heterozygotes, or carriers, for the CF gene. A simple punnet square will reveal that of the four possible genotypes one can have in the offspring (of those individuals carrying a recessive disorder), one in four will have the double dose, or be homozygous for the recessive. Two individuals will have a single dose of the recessive gene and be carriers, and one will be normal. Since in CF the carriers are not clinically affected, there would be three normal individuals possible in the offspring. Two of those three will be carriers, hence the 2/3 proportion.

24 and 25. The answers are: 24-B, 25-C. *(Hepatitis B virus)* Patients who have a history of hepatitis infection must be followed up for signs and symptoms of a chronic hepatitis infection (one that lasts more than 6 months). Chronic hepatitis may result from hepatitis B viral infection, hepatitis non-A, non-B viral infections, drugs, toxins, and inborn errors of metabolism. Clinical manifestations may be nonexistent, and laboratory manifestations may be minimal, or both may reveal progressive liver failure.

26. The answer is B. *(Diabetes-associated renal disease)* Membranous glomerulonephritis is characterized by electron-dense deposits along the epithelial side of the glomerular basement membrane. The renal pathology observed in long-term diabetic patients includes capillary basement membrane thickening, diffuse glomerulosclerosis (a diffuse increase in mesangial matrix and cellularity), and Kimmelstiel–Wilson syndrome (also known as nodular glomerulosclerosis or intercapillary glomerulosclerosis; the lesions consist of hyaline masses situated in the periphery of the glomerulus). Infiltration of glomeruli with polymorphonuclear leukocytes and monocytes is common in poststreptococcal glomerulonephritis.

27–29. The answers are: 27-B, 28-C, 29-C. *(Medical genetics and Down syndrome)* The infant has trisomy 21 (Down syndrome), which occurs by nondisjunction during cell division. Developmental assessment or an electroencephalogram would contribute to the physical assessment of the patient but would not be diagnostic of the condition. Diagnosis is best made by karyotype. The condition is not a mucopolysaccharidosis; therefore, a urine spot test would not be appropriate. Case studies of families in which trisomy 21 has occurred show that their risk of nondisjunction occurring again is about 1%, or 1 in 100.

30–35. The answers are: 30-B, 31-D, 32-A, 33-E, 34-D, 35-A. *(Adverse drug reactions; chemotherapeutic and cardiovascular pharmacology)* Gentamicin, an aminoglycoside, is used for the treatment of infections caused by gram-negative bacteria. It has no anticancer activity. Adriamycin, cisplatin (cis-diamminedichloroplatinum), and cyclophosphamide are frequently used in combination for the treatment of ovarian cancer. Melphalan is an alkylating agent that is also useful in the treatment of this malignancy.

Cefoxitin is a second-generation cephalosporin with a broad spectrum of activity against both gram-negative and gram-positive bacteria, including β-lactamase–producing organisms. Cefoxitin should be used because the patient has been treated with antineoplastic drugs and may be at risk for infection due to immunosuppression. Most cephalosporins, including cefoxitin, cannot be administered orally and have no selective distribution. They have no antineoplastic activity and cannot be mixed with aminoglycosides.

Antimicrobial drugs, such as penicillins and, less frequently, cephalosporins, can cause type I allergic reactions with resultant anaphylaxis, urticaria, and extrinsic asthma. This is due to the release of histamine and other noncytotoxic mediators from basophilic leukocytes and tissue mast cells.

Cefoxitin acts as a hapten often in complex with a protein and causes the proliferation of lymphoid B cells that produce IgE antibodies. This sensitizes basophils or mast cells, which when re-exposed can bind the antigens leading to the release of noncytotoxic substances such as histamine and leukotrienes. All of the immediate physiologic and pathologic effects described in this patient can ensue.

Bronchoconstriction is induced by the release of histamine, and a major therapeutic goal is to reduce bronchoconstriction. Epinephrine blocks the release of mediators from mast cells and basophils, while dexamethasone inhibits the proliferation of IgE-producing cells and blocks helper–T-cell function, in addition to its anti-inflammatory effect. Diphenhydramine competitively blocks histamine actions at H_1 receptors that would otherwise cause bronchoconstriction.

The cardiovascular changes occurring during a type I allergic drug reaction often are secondary to hypoxia due to bronchoconstriction, especially if there is underlying ischemic heart disease. There is also some evidence that the heart may become sensitized to IgE-mediated antigens. There is no evidence for direct cardiovascular or vagal effects of cefoxitin, and infiltration of endogenous cells into the heart musculature is not seen.

36. The answer is A. *(Hematopoietic-lymphoreticular system)* Reed-Sternberg cells are diaganostic for Hodgkin's lymphoma. The Philadelphia chromosome and decreased quanities of leukocyte alkaline phosphatase are commonly observed in chronic myelogenous leukemia. Auer rods are most often seen in increased numbers in acute myelogenous or myelomonocytic leukemia.

37. The answer is E. *(Serum sickness)* The most likely cause of this situation is the deposition of antigen–antibody complexes made of horse proteins and human immunoglobulins. Drops in complement levels signal immune complex reactions. The amount of venom protein alone is insufficient to cause an appreciable precipitate. Delayed and anaphylactic reactions would not cause joint pain or dark urine.

38. The answer is D. *(Tumor immunology)* Mutation of the tumor-associated antigen gene, complement depletion as a result of the liver metastasis, and the appearance of antibodies to mouse immunoglobulins are all valid explanations of the problem posed in the question. The amount of antigen on the tumor cell, rather than the serum levels, is important.

39. The answer is B. *(Nonsteroidal anti-inflammatory drugs)* The major adverse effect of aspirin is gastrointestinal bleeding. Inhibition of local cytoprotective arachidonic acid metabolites (prostaglandin E_2 and prostacyclin) in the gastric mucosa contributes to this adverse effect and can be offset by simultaneously using exogenous synthetic prostanoids. In addition, aspirin has a direct irritating effect on the mucosa. Nonsteroidal anti-inflammatory agents in general have little effect on lipoxygenase activity but do affect cyclooxygenase. In particular, aspirin is an irreversible inhibitor of this enzyme in platelets (and other cell types) by acetylating the α-amino group of the terminal serine. This irreversible inhibition has significant implications in that platelet function will not be restored to normal until a new enzyme has been synthesized. Aspirin has little effect on normal body temperature but reduces abnormally elevated body temperatures secondary to alterations in central thermoregulation.

40. The answer is B. *(Inflammation)* Infiltration by polymorphonuclear leukocytes is a major characteristic of acute inflammation, not classic chronic inflammation. Typical causes of chronic inflammation include progression from acute inflammation, repeated bouts of acute inflammation, and persistent low-grade inflammation that does not progress to classic acute inflammation. Macrophages are the essential component of chronic inflammation because they produce substances that mediate the inflammatory response, including chemotactic factors, complement components, and growth factors.

41. The answer is D. *(Gonococcal salpingitis)* For all practical purposes, the patient is cured. However, women who have suffered from gonorrhea are a population at risk of future complications, such as subsequent episodes of pelvic inflammatory disease, infertility, and ectopic pregnancy.

42. The answer is D. *(Hypokalemia and action of diuretics)* Loop diuretics, such as furosemide, act primarily on the thick segment of the ascending limb of the loop of Henle, abolishing transepithelial potential difference and, thereby, inhibiting transport of NaCl out of the tubule into the interstitium. In addition, more solute is delivered to the distal portions of the nephron where water reabsorption is reduced further by osmotic effect. By a poorly understood subsidiary effect, furosemide increases renal blood flow without affecting glomerular filtration and, thus, an additional oncotic stimulus presents more solute and water to the tubular system. The presentation of large amounts of Na^+ to the collecting tubules results in excretion of K^+ and H^+, causing profound hypokalemia. The K^+ loss and the relative hypovolemia stimulate H^+ secretion and HCO_3^- generation. Intracellular K^+ is also exchanged in the body for H^+, further affecting metabolic alkalosis. Increased NaCl excretion also causes loss of Ca^{2+} and Mg^{2+}. Dietary supplementation of K^+ or the use of concomitant K^+-sparing agents, like spironolactone, are used to offset the hypokalemia and metabolic alkalosis caused by furosemide.

43 and 44. The answers are: 43-C, 44-C. *(Pulmonary mechanics and pharmacotherapy)* Bronchial asthma is the most likely diagnosis of the condition of the 10-year-old child described in the question, based on the history and the reversible changes after administration of a bronchodilator. The most common therapy for mild childhood asthma is now cromolyn sodium (Intal). Cromolyn appears to work by interfering with the immunologically mediated, and perhaps nonimmunologically mediated, release of biologically active endogenous substances from mast and other cells that cause bronchoconstriction, airway edema, and hypersecretion of mucus. Although histamine is presumably one of these endogenous substances, antihistamines do not have a role in the therapy of asthma except for reducing some symptoms, such as rhinitis. Propranolol is contraindicated in asthmatics. Although anti-inflammatory therapy is an important aspect of treating asthma, aspirin may lead to a nonimmunologically mediated anaphylactoid reaction and is not considered appropriate prophylactic therapy for asthma. However, corticosteroids are an important pharmacotherapeutic regimen for significant asthmatic conditions. Neostigmine is a cholinesterase inhibitor and may be expected to exacerbate symptoms by enhancing cholinergic transmission within the bronchial smooth muscle and airways. Other common agents used for asthma include β-adrenergic agonists, phosphodiesterase inhibitors (with adenosine receptor antagonist effects), anticholinergic agents, and glucocorticosteroids.

Stimulation of irritant receptors leads to reflex bronchoconstriction via a vagal reflex. Indeed, normal resting tone is set by the parasympathetic nervous system, and some aspects of hyperreactive airways disease (asthma) are thought to involve a relatively high influence of vagal tone at the expense of sympathetic efferent bronchodilator activity. The intercostal and phrenic nerves are important nerves to accessory muscle and the diaphragm, respectively.

45. The answer is B. *(Medical genetics and Tay-Sachs disease)* The frequency of the Tay-Sachs gene is 1/30. The frequency of carriers of Tay-Sachs can be calculated from the Hardy-Weinberg equation, where carrier frequency is equal to $2pq$. The gene frequency (q) can be calculated by taking the square root of the incidence (q^2); the square root of $1/3600 = 1/60$. The value of p is equal to $1 - q$; $60/60 - 1/60 = 59/60$. In most cases of rare diseases, p becomes equal to 1 and the carrier frequency becomes $2q$; $2 \times 1/60 = 1/30$.

46. The answer is E. *(Recurrent urinary tract infections)* Longitudinal studies have shown that bacteriuria in women susceptible to urinary tract infections is preceded by colonization of the vaginal introitus with the responsible organism from the rectal flora.

47. The answer is E. *(Gas exchange and partial pressure of oxygen)* The change in cabin air pressure will cause a modest reduction in arterial Po_2. The partial pressure of a gas is proportional to the fractional concentration of the gas and total gas pressure. Predictably, Po_2 would decrease from the normal range of 97 to 100 mm Hg to about 67 mm Hg following decreases in alveolar Po_2. This decrease is partially due to water vapor pressure, which remains constant at 47 mm Hg, and Pco_2, which may decrease slightly due to stimulation from ventilation. This modest decline in Po_2 would not be associated with a decrease in oxygen saturation of arterial hemoglobin. A compensatory response would shift the oxyhemoglobin dissociation curve to the right, due to the production of 2,3-diphosphoglycerate (2,3-DPG); however, this response usually takes more time than the average plane flight.

48. The answer is D. *(Delayed-type hypersensitivity reactions)* The reaction observed was most likely caused by CD4+ T cells. It is a delayed reaction, demonstrating that the T cells are working fine; therefore, the patient could neither lack all T-cell–mediated immune function nor suffer from DiGeorge syndrome. Sensitization has already occurred, so that subsequent exposure would produce symptoms faster than the primary reaction.

49. The answer is A. *(Rheumatoid arthritis)* Subcutaneous nodules may be present in rheumatoid arthritis, and can be distinguished from the similar-appearing, urate-containing gouty tophi. Involvement of the distal interphalangeal joints is almost never seen in rheumatoid arthritis. Rheumatoid arthritis almost always results in symmetrical, multiple joint involvement, whereas osteoarthritis often presents in a single joint or as asymmetrical joint involvement. Rheumatoid factor is a 19S IgM directed against the Fc fragment of IgG.

50–54. The answers are: 50-B, 51-B, 52-B, 53-C, 54-A. *(Mechanism of action of antineoplastic agents)* This is a classic case of cisplatin-induced renal toxicity. As with most renal toxins, the region usually affected is the highly metabolically active proximal tubules. Mannitol is added to the treatment regimen to reduce the transit time of cisplatin in the proximal tubules of the kidneys and, thus, reduce the renal toxicity caused by cisplatin. Cisplatin generally causes little myelosuppression, although it may cause transient leukopenia and thrombocytopenia.

Bleomycin was added to the regimen because of its activity in squamous carcinoma of the neck. The most serious adverse effect of the drug is pulmonary toxicity. Damage to the kidney, as occurred in this case with cisplatin, can lead to a marked decrease in the excretion of bleomycin and, thus, increases its plasma half-life and its toxicity to the lungs.

The mechanism of action of cisplatin is thought to be covalent interaction with DNA. Cisplatin is a neutral coordination metal complex that undergoes rapid nonenzymatic aquation to form DNA-reactive species of the drug once inside the cell. This is thought to block DNA transcription and replication. Cisplatin can react with RNA and proteins, but this is not thought to result in significant cell death.

The mechanism of action of bleomycin involves fragmentation of both single and double DNA strands. It has nucleotide-sequence specificity and, thus, it acts much like a restriction enzyme. This reaction requires O_2 and Fe^{2+} and is due to noncovalent binding of a drug–O_2–Fe^{2+} complex to DNA.

55. The answer is B. *(Hematology and neutrophils)* The cell in this blood smear probably is a neutrophil. The Barr body is found only in females and contains an inactive (condensed) X chromosome. The Barr body, or drumstick chromosome, is found in approximately 3% of neutrophils.

56. The answer is A. *(Diagnosis of myelodysplastic syndrome)* Clinically persistent and unexplained cytopenias associated with morphologically abnormal differentiation in bone marrow precursors defines preleukemia, often referred to as the myelodysplastic syndrome. Many of these individuals will have bone marrow blast percentages of < 5%, and patients suffer from complications of bone marrow failure such as bleeding, infection, and anemia. Others will show an increase in bone marrow blasts between 5% and 30% and have a higher propensity to develop frank acute myeloid leukemia, particularly at the higher levels. Bone marrow blasts > 30% defines acute leukemia. Cytogenetic changes, if present in myelodysplastic syndrome, are similar to those observed with acute myeloid leukemia, such as an extra chromosome 8, loss of chromosome 5 or 7, or loss of the long arm of chromosome 5 or 7. Despite megaloblastoid morphologic changes, symptoms do not resolve with treatment for megaloblastic anemia. It is rare for chronic myelogenous leukemia to present with a low white cell and platelet count and bone marrow dyspoiesis.

57. The answer is A. *(Viral structure and neutrophils)* In viruses that have a segmented genome, each RNA piece encodes at least one protein. The fact that the mRNA (defined as positive-sense or positive-polarity RNA) isolated from infected cells hybridizes to virion genomic RNA means that the latter must be negative-sense; thus distractor (C) is wrong. Negative-sense RNA molecules are never infectious by themselves because they require an attached virus-encoded transcriptase to enter the cell with them; hence distractor (B) is incorrect. Viral RNA genomes are replicated by virus-specific enzymes because cellular polymerases synthesize RNA only from DNA templates.

58. The answer is E. *(Neuroleptic agents)* Chlorpromazine is a neuroleptic (antipsychotic) agent that is a dopamine receptor antagonist as well as having many other pharmacologic effects (e.g., antimuscarinic, α-adrenergic receptor antagonism, antihistaminic). In 15% to 20% of older patients taking the drug for schizophrenic disorders, a poorly understood syndrome of tardive dyskinesia occurs that is not readily reversible even after stopping chlorpromazine. The syndrome is typified by repetitive, involuntary movements of the oral–facial area. Widespread choreoathetosis and dystonia may also occur. The mechanism is poorly understood but may be secondary to excess function of dopamine due to compensatory changes in the basal ganglia. The seizure-like symptoms (acute dystonia), motor restlessness (akathisia), and parkinsonism are all acute changes. Similarly, acute orthostatic hypotension may occur secondary to α-adrenergic blockade. In general, the extrapyramidal effects of antipsychotics may be minimized with some drugs that have significant antimuscarinic activity, such as clozapine.

59. The answer is A. *(Malaria)* Of the major diseases with geographic relevance, malaria is one of the few that can be rapidly life-threatening. The other diseases listed (i.e., chronic Chagas disease, amebic dysentery, mucocutaneous leishmaniasis, and giardiasis) are either chronically debilitating or subpatent in nature. Amebic dysentery and giardiasis are not life-threatening conditions, and it is not necessary to determine the species for treatment of either. No effective treatment exists for chronic Chagas disease, so rapid diagnosis is not essential. While determination of the species of *Leishmania* is useful in distinguishing cutaneous and mucocutaneous leishmaniasis in terms of treatment, both are long-term infections and not life-threatening.

60. The answer is C. *(Adverse effects of corticosteroids)* Long-term use of corticosteroids suppresses the patient's own response to infection or injury and greatly limits its overall usefulness. Exogenous steroids inhibit the patient's capacity to synthesize corticosteroids, and thus, acute withdrawal may precipitate adrenal insufficiency. Corticosteroids, like dexamethasone, are relatively free of mineralocorticoid effects. However, if given in large doses, they can cause iatrogenic Cushing's syndrome that includes a hyperglycemic effect. Although the mechanism by which steroids produce any of the above responses is unclear, it appears that they induce the synthesis of lipocortin, which, in turn, inhibits phospholipase A_2 activity.

61. The answer is E. *(Membrane physiology)* Application of acetylcholine (ACh) or vagal stimulation decreases the slope of phase 4 of a slow fiber (or pacemaker cell) that is likely to be found in the sinoatrial or atrioventricular nodal tissue. This is due to increased permeability to K^+ and causes a decrease in heart rate in situ. Fast fibers like those found in non-nodal atrial or ventricular tissue have a rapid depolarization (phase 0) due to the opening of fast Na^+ channels, followed by a plateau (phase 2) secondary to the opening of slow Ca^{2+} channels.

62. The answer is B. *(Reproductive physiology)* Trisomy 21 (Down syndrome), a major cause of mental retardation, does not have an associated increased incidence of cryptorchidism. Cryptorchidism is failure of the testicles to descend into the scrotum and is the most common congenital anomaly (present in 0.3% to 0.5% of all male births). Most cases are idiopathic, but other causes include mechanical abnormalities (e.g., short spermatic cord, narrow inguinal canal), hormonal abnormalities (e.g., deficiency of luteinizing hormone–releasing hormone), and genetic abnormalities (e.g., trisomy 13).

63–66. The answers are: 63-B, 64-D, 65-B, 66-C. *(Acid–base physiology)* The blood findings indicate that this patient has a respiratory alkalosis, an acid–base disturbance characterized by increased arterial pH (or decreased $[H^+]$), decreased $Paco_2$ (hypocapnia), and decreased plasma $[HCO_3^-]$. It should be noted that both $[H^+]$ and $[HCO_3^-]$ are decreased in this patient, which is consistent with the axiom that $[H^+]$ and $[HCO_3^-]$ change in the same direction in respiratory acid–base imbalances. The decline in $[HCO_3^-]$ indicates that renal compensation has begun.

In alkalotic states, the $[HCO_3^-]/S \times Pco_2$ ratio exceeds the normal 20:1, due to either an increase in $[HCO_3^-]$ (metabolic alkalosis) or a decrease in Pco_2 (respiratory alkalosis). S is a solubility constant. The normal ratio of 20:1 is derived as

$$\frac{[HCO_3^-]}{S \times Pco_2} = \frac{24 \text{ mmol/L}}{0.03 \times 40 \text{ mm Hg}} = \frac{24 \text{ mmol/L}}{1.2 \text{ mmol/L}} = \frac{20}{1}$$

In this alkalotic patient, the $[HCO_3^-]/S \times Pco_2$ ratio is 30:1. This ratio can be determined by substituting the patient's blood data into the above equation, as

$$\frac{[HCO_3^-]}{S \times Pco_2} = \frac{22.5 \text{ mmol/L}}{0.03 \times 25 \text{ mm Hg}} = \frac{22.5 \text{ mmol/L}}{0.75 \text{ mmol/L}} = \frac{30}{1}$$

The total CO_2 content for this patient is approximately 23 mmol/L. Total CO_2 equals the sum of all forms of CO_2 in the blood (i.e., HCO_3^-, H_2CO_3, dissolved CO_2, and CO_2 bound to proteins). Dissolved CO_2 content ($[CO_2]$) is calculated as

$$[CO_2] = 0.03 \times P_{CO_2}$$
$$= 0.03 \times 40 \text{ mm Hg}$$
$$= 1.2 \text{ mmol/L}$$

Since $[H_2CO_3]$ is negligible, the total CO_2 content normally exceeds the $[HCO_3^-]$ by 1.2 mmol/L and, therefore, equals 25.2 mmol/L when normal plasma $[HCO_3^-]$ and P_{CO_2} values exist, as

$$\text{total } CO_2 \text{ content} = [HCO_3^-] + (S \times P_{CO_2})$$
$$= 24 \text{ mmol/L} + 1.2 \text{ mmol/L}$$
$$= 25.2 \text{ mmol/L}$$

Total CO_2 content is decreased in respiratory alkalosis. From this patient's blood data, the CO_2 content is calculated as

$$\text{total } CO_2 \text{ content} = [HCO_3^-] + (S \times P_{CO_2})$$
$$= 22.5 \text{ mmol/L} + 0.75 \text{ mmol/L}$$
$$= 23.25 \text{ mmol/L}$$

Respiratory alkalosis decreases the renal reabsorption of HCO_3^-, causing a transient HCO_3^- diuresis and a decline in net acid secretion. Since the major change in respiratory alkalosis is a decrease in P_{aCO_2}, the compensation will be in the alternate variable (kidney) and in the same direction as the primary event. Thus, there is a decline in plasma $[HCO_3^-]$, which is indicative of a partial renal response (i.e., increased HCO_3^- excretion).

67. The answer is A. *(Pancreatic islet cell function and insulin-dependent diabetes mellitus type I therapy)* Sulfonylureas and other oral hypoglycemics are contraindicated in insulin-dependent diabetes (IDD) because of lack of functioning pancreatic β cells in IDD. Insulin therapy to maintain blood glucose levels within a physiologic range is a symptomatic approach to the treatment of IDD. Blood glucose levels are routinely monitored, and insulin is adjusted to maintain the blood glucose levels. A frequent side effect is hypoglycemia, which is best treated by ingestion of carbohydrates. Some patients who still maintain a normal response to glucagon benefit by injection of glucagon for this crisis as well. Although recombinant forms of insulin have reduced insulin insensitivity due to an immune response, this problem still persists. Apparently the source of the hormone (animal versus human) is not the only determinant of antigenicity.

68–70. The answers are: 68-D, 69-A, 70-E. *(Mechanics of respiration)* One of the simplest and most useful tests of lung function is forced expiration. The spirometric recordings in the figure that accompanies the question are from a normal subject, A, and the patient, B, who has obstructive lung disease. The low flow rate over most of the forced expiration (as estimated by the tangent to the spirometric volume–time tracing) is partly due to decreased elastic recoil of the lung. In obstructive lung disease, forced expiratory volume in 1 second (FEV_1), forced vital capacity (FVC), and FEV_1/FVC are all reduced due to airway obstruction (i.e., mucus in the lumen, thickening of the airway wall), and the expiratory time is prolonged.

Many patients with chronic bronchitis tend to retain CO_2 at some time in their disease (either advanced or during exercise). An important contributing factor is their increased work of breathing secondary to airway obstruction. Apparently, these patients attempt to conserve oxygen expenditure by not adequately increasing ventilation at the cost of an elevated arterial P_{CO_2}. These patients have a modest increase in physiologic dead space, and this tends to reduce arterial P_{CO_2}. They also have a large physiologic shunt (high blood flow to poorly ventilated areas of lung) that tends to make them hypoxemic but has little effect on arterial P_{CO_2}.

The physiologic and clinical description of the patient is consistent with a diagnosis of chronic bronchitis. A histopathologic hallmark of this disorder is hypertrophy of bronchial mucosal glands. Indeed, this pathologic change, along with remodeling of the submucosa, has given rise to a morphogenic description of the disorder and a quantitative index of the disease (Reid index). Caseating necrosis is a critical pathologic change in tuberculosis. Noncaseating granuloma and thickening of the interstitium are consistent with restrictive disorders, including sarcoidosis and diffuse interstitial pulmonary fibrosis, respectively. Plexiform pulmonary arteriopathy is an important characteristic of primary (and secondary) pulmonary hypertension and, in general, is not a hallmark of chronic bronchitis.

71. The answer is D. *(Efficacy of zidovudine)* Zidovudine (ZDV) is currently the most important agent available for the palliation of AIDS. ZDV is phosphorylated to a deoxynucleoside derivative, which inhibits viral RNA-dependent DNA polymerase. Its selectivity is a function of its specificity for reverse transcriptase compared to human DNA polymerase. Granulocytopenia and anemia occur in up to 45% of treated patients, and resistance does occur to the drug after prolonged therapy. ZDV delays the development of signs and symptoms of AIDS in patients who are asymptomatic and improves the clinical symptoms of patients with AIDS at most stages in their disease. Thus, the incidence of opportunistic infections decreases, and there are some improvements in neurologic deficits, AIDS-associated thrombocytopenia, psoriasis, and lymphocytic interstitial pneumonia.

72 and 73. The answers are: 72-A, 73-C. *(Pharmacokinetics)* The volume of distribution (V_d) is the ratio of the amount injected to the extrapolated concentration (C_0) at time zero. Since equal amounts of X, Y, and Z were injected, V_d is inversely related to C_0. Therefore, X and Z have an identical V_d, and V_d Y > V_d X or V_d Z. Clearance is proportional to the ratio of V_d to half-time ($t_{1/2}$). Since $V_d Y > V_d X$, clearance of Y > clearance of X. Since $t_{1/2}Z < t_{1/2}X$ (which is identical to $t_{1/2}Y$), clearance of Z < clearace of X.

The time to reach steady state is purely a function of $t_{1/2}$. Since $t_{1/2} Z > t_{1/2} X$ or $t_{1/2} Y$, it will take Z longer to reach a steady state than either X or Y. However, X and Y will reach a steady state at precisely the same time. The steady-state concentration (C_{ss}) is a function of the ratio of infused rate to clearance. The infused rates are constant, so C_{ss} is inversely related to clearance. Since clearance of Y > clearance of X or clearance of Z, then steady-state concentrations will be [Z] > [X] > [Y].

74. The answer is E. *(Urinary tract infection therapy)* Penicillin G is the treatment of choice. It is inexpensive, and it is a broad-spectrum antibiotic at urinary concentrations. The serum levels are so low that it is unlikely to alter the natural bacterial flora of the host.

75. The answer is A. *(Capillary physiology)* If the permeability of the lung remains constant, increased left atrial pressure could lead to pulmonary interstitial edema. Factors that tend to elevate microvascular pressure will increase the Starling forces that favor net filtration of fluid. Left atrial hypertension caused by many factors, including mitral valve disease and left heart failure, is a common cause of nonpermeability (or cardiogenic) pulmonary edema. Decreases in right atrial pressure reduce fluid flow across the lungs by reducing backpressure to the drainage of pulmonary lymph or, more likely, will have little effect on lung fluid balance. A decrease, not increase, in circulating proteins would cause edema. Since lymphatics have unidirectional valves, increasing the pumping action of these vessels tends to drive fluid out of the organ.

76. The answer is C. *(Platelet homeostasis)* Examination of the peripheral blood smear must never be overlooked when evaluating a patient for thrombocytopenia. Unreported abnormalities of the red cells may offer a clue to the etiology, or occasionally one may find a discrepancy between the number of platelets seen on the smear and that found by the automated count, as in pseudothrombocytopenia, where clumping of platelets in a specific anticoagulant (usually EDTA) results in marked underestimation of the count.

77. The answer is B. *(Type II diabetes mellitus)* There is often a 90% to 100% concordance rate in identical twins (i.e., both twins are nearly always affected), demonstrating that environmental factors are not usually important in the pathogenesis of type II diabetes mellitus (type II DM). Other features observed in type II DM include obesity, normal or increased blood insulin levels, and insulin resistance. This is in contrast to type I DM in which the onset of disease is in the first or second decade of life and insulin levels are severely depressed due to destruction of islet beta cells. In this case, there is only an approximate 50% concordance in identical twins, and there is an apparent linkage of the disease with human leukocyte antigen D (HLA-D). This linkage is thought to provide a predisposition of the beta cells to destructive environmental factors.

78. The answer is D. *(Hyperthyroidism)* Tachycardia is a common clinical manifestation of hyperthyroidism. Hyperthyroidism is most commonly caused by an autoimmune disorder. It results in an enlarged gland (goiter) with increased circulating levels of free thyroxine. These increased levels suppress thyroid-stimulating hormone (TSH) secretion so that it will not respond to exogenous thyrotropin-releasing hormone (TRH). In addition to important signs such as exophthalmos and infiltrative dermatitis, much of the clinical syndrome is secondary to overactivity of the adrenergic nervous system. Accordingly, heart rate is usually increased and other metabolic and central activities are also stimulated.

79 and 80. The answers are: 79-B, 80-C. *(Urine output)* The diuresis in the 76-year-old man described in the question is the result of excessive urea, which acts as an osmotic diuretic, combined with volume overload owing to the obstruction. The postobstructive diuresis is characterized by a decreased glomerular filtration rate (GFR), increased tubular permeability, and a lack of responsiveness to both antidiuretic hormone and aldosterone.

81. The answer is D. *(Facial nerves and vessels)* The pterygopalatine fossa contains the pterygopalatine ganglion, the maxillary division of the trigeminal nerve (CN V), and branches of the maxillary artery, including the infraorbital artery. The pterygoid venous plexus, however, does not lie within the fossa but instead is closely associated with the lateral pterygoid muscle.

82. The answer is C. *(Diagnosis of acute rheumatic fever)* The diagnosis of acute rheumatic fever must fulfill the modified Jones criteria; this requires the presence of at least two major criteria or one major and two minor criteria plus supportive evidence of a prior streptococcal infection. The major clinical manifestations, according to these criteria, include carditis, polyarthritis, chorea, erythema marginatum, and subcutaneous nodules; the minor criteria include prior history of acute rheumatic fever or rheumatic heart disease, arthralgia, fever, elevated serum acute-phase reactants, and prolonged PR interval on an electrocardiogram (ECG). Supportive evidence of a prior streptococcal infection includes increased serum antistreptococcal antibodies, positive throat culture, and recent history of scarlet fever.

83. The answer is E. *(Serologic markers for hepatitis B virus)* The presence of hepatitis B surface antigen (HBsAg), hepatitis B e antigen (HBeAg), anti-HBc antibodies, and anti-HBe antibodies indicates that an individual has already been exposed to hepatitis B virus (HBV) and thus would not be a candidate for vaccine. Hepatitis B vaccine contains triple-activated and purified HBV surface antigen (HBsAg) taken from carrier serum. Three doses administered over 6 months results in the production of anti-HBs antibodies in the patient. Protection approaches nearly 100% after three doses.

84. The answer is A. *(Retroviruses, lentiviruses, and oncoviruses)* The human retroviruses, HTLV-I, HTLV-II, and HTLV-III (HIV) do not fully transform cells into malignant or cancer cells alone. In fact, HIV is able to lyse helper T-lymphocytes under certain conditions, which leads to the immunosuppression associated with AIDS. HTLV-I and HTLV-II are oncoviruses, whereas HIV is a lentivirus. The β-type particle morphology is characteristic only of the mouse mammary tumor virus. One of the most important distinguishing features of human retroviruses is the relatively large number of genes they possess in addition to *gag, pol,* and *env.*

85. The answer is D. *(Tumor pathology)* Although malignant transformation of a benign neoplasm may occur, it is rare. More often, fatality due to a benign neoplasm is the result of interference with the function of a vital organ. Bleeding due to the expansive growth of a benign tumor is a less likely event than is bleeding due to the invasion and ulceration of tissues or to the infiltration and eventual rupture of vessels by a malignant tumor. Occasionally, multifocal benign neoplasms are found, but this is not a likely cause of death. Any neoplasm can invoke an immune response.

86. The answer is A. *(Anatomy of lymphatics)* Breast cancer that presents as a lump in the lower medial quadrant probably signifies initial involvement of the internal thoracic nodes. Lymphatic vessels from the medial half of the breast pierce the second, third, and fourth intercostal spaces to drain into lymph nodes along the internal thoracic artery. Lymph from the lateral breast flows to anterior axillary nodes. Occasionally, involvement of supraclavicular nodes may accompany invasion of superior mammary lobes.

87. The answer is B. *(pH partitioning)* A weak base such as phenobarbital tends to be in its ionized form at a higher pH. Therefore, alkalinizing the urine with $NaHCO_3$ has the desired effect of hastening renal elimination. In addition, urine flow increases in an alkaline situation, further increasing the amount of phenobarbital that is eliminated. Alkalinization of plasma will also tend to move un-ionized phenobarbital out of the central nervous system (CNS) and into the plasma, by creating a transient gradient in which movement can occur. Phenobarbital and other barbiturates tend to induce P450 enzymes, which should aid the elimination of these drugs. However, the induction of P450 enzymes is somewhat slower than desired in an emergency situation.

88. The answer is D. *(Immunogenetics)* The results of the HLA typing for this particular case show that the mother is homozygous for HLA-A1. The haplotypes of the mother are A1/B5 and A1/B7. The real father's haplotypes are A3/B12 and A9/B17; therefore, the alleged father is probably the real father of both children. Child 1 is A1/B5 and A3/B12 and does not share haplotypes with child 2, who is A1/B7 and A9/B17.

89. The answer is D. *(Neurotransmitters and parkinsonism)* Important pathophysiologic changes in parkinsonism include a decrease in the level of dopamine and degeneration of dopaminergic neurons in the nigrostriatal tract with an increase in cholinergic transmission. Accordingly, current therapy is aimed at restoring a more normal balance either by increasing dopamine levels in the central nervous system (CNS) [with levodopa and semicarbidopa therapy, monoamine oxidase (MAO) inhibition, or even transplantation of dopamine-secreting cells into the brain] or inhibiting excessive cholinergic transmission with antimuscarinic drugs (atropine). Prolonging the half-life of acetylcholine (ACh) is likely to result in an exacerbation of the symptoms.

90 and 91. The answers are: 90-C, 91-B. *(Cardiac mechanics and congestive heart failure)* The major signs of congestive heart failure are fatigue and dyspnea. Vascular congestion as confirmed by physical examination (i.e., neck veins, rales) and third heart sounds due to abnormally high diastolic flow to a normal ventricle or normal flow into a dilated ventricle are also consistent with congestive heart failure. The enlarged cardiac silhouette with pulmonary vascular markings is strongly suggestive of left-sided heart failure. Neither the heart rate nor blood pressure is elevated significantly enough to consider this a malignant arrhythmia or emergency hypertensive crisis.

In the control subject (X), end-diastolic pressure is low, and ejection is well-maintained during systole. In the failing heart, end-diastolic pressure and volume are greatly elevated, and ejection is poorly maintained (stroke volume is reduced). Digitalis (Y) exerts a positive inotropic effect by inhibiting Na^+-K^+ ATPase and indirectly elevating intracellular Ca^+. The effect is to decrease diastolic pressures and volumes and increase stroke volume.

92. The answer is E. *(DNA structure)* An analysis of chromosomal DNA using the Southern blot technique starts with the cleavage of the DNA with restriction enzymes followed by electrophoresis on agarose gel, which separates the DNA fragments by fragment size. The DNA fragments are transferred to a sheet of nitrocellulose by a flow of buffer (blotting). The fragments bind to the nitrocellulose, creating a replica of the pattern of DNA fragments on the gel, which is visualized by autoradiography.

93. The answer is B. *(Type II immunity)* Erythroblastosis fetalis is a hemolytic anemia in the neonate — a classic type II reaction in which maternal IgG antibodies cross the placenta and usually attach to Rh antigen. This opsonization of fetal red blood cells causes lysis by complement fixation or antibody-dependent, cell-mediated cytotoxicity. The lysis can produce varying degrees of anemia and jaundice. Erythroblastosis fetalis manifests itself as a mild to severe disease and, in some cases, can cause death.

94. The answer is D. *(Sodium channels and local anesthetics)* Local anesthetics block Na^+ channels and decrease conductance of Na^+, thereby inhibiting depolarization and normal conduction of action potentials. Small, myelinated nerve fibers are most sensitive, and differential sensitivity explains preferential blockade for pain sensation as opposed to other sensory modalities. Lidocaine is highly lipid-soluble and may cause convulsions if sufficient amounts are delivered to the brain. By affecting Na^+ channels in cardiovascular tissue, dysrhythmia and decreased contractility may ensue. The ester anesthetics, such as procaine, are substrates for plasma cholinesterases, whereas lidocaine is more slowly metabolized in the liver. Local anesthetics such as lidocaine are useful for more widespread blockade of neurotransmission after direct placement in spinal fluid.

95. The answer is D. *(Musculature of the back)* The levator costarum muscles, which connect each vertebral transverse process to the rib below, would not be encountered in the midaxillary line. All three intercostal muscles (i.e., external intercostal, internal intercostal, and transverse thoracis muscles) are present at the posterior midaxillary line. Also, the serratus anterior muscle is encountered at rib seven as it passes from its origin at the upper eight ribs to insert into the scapula.

96. The answer is A. *(Allotypic markers on immunoglobulin)* The patient's serum blocks the anti-G1m(a) and anti-G1m(x) reactions and, therefore, must contain molecules that interact with anti-allotypic antibody reagents. The other reactions are not blocked; therefore, there are no allotypic antibodies of that type in the patient's serum.

97. The answer is B. *(Pulmonary mechanics)* Compliance is defined as change in volume over change in pressure. The steeper the curves of the static volume–pressure relationships shown in the figure, the more compliant the lungs are. A compliant, or flabby, lung is typical of emphysema, where recoil pressures are lower at any given lung volume and the functional residual capacity tends to be higher. In contrast, a fibrotic, stiff lung (subject C) has decreased compliance and increased elastic recoil and tends to have a lower functional residual capacity. This increased elastic recoil pulls the chest wall in until the outward recoil of the chest wall equals (but is opposite) the inward recoil of the lung, hence lowering functional residual capacity.

98. The answer is D. *(Vaccines as applied to AIDS)* Of the vaccination procedures listed, the one most likely to be tested by the Food and Drug Administration (FDA) is the procedure that uses a human monoclonal antibody that reacts with the intact CD4 (T4) receptor. Antibodies that react with CD4 should "look like" the portion of human immunodeficiency virus (HIV) that reacts with the CD4 receptor. Therefore, the vaccinated person should make an antibody to the human monoclonal antibody, which may be protective against HIV.

99. The answer is B. *(Gerontology)* The selectivity of the deficit makes a supraforaminal lesion and a peripheral neuropathy impossible. We are not told if position sense is impaired: If it is, the posterior column of the spinal cord becomes a possibility, but an isolated vibratory deficit can occur as a normal aging change. The practical point is that when diminished vibratory sensation is encountered, position sense must be tested carefully.

100. The answer is B. *(Microcirculation)* There is decreased protein content of the edema fluid in cardiogenic edema as opposed to noncardiogenic pulmonary edema. The pulmonary endothelium is essentially undamaged in cardiogenic edema, so the pulmonary transudate consists of a filtrate of low protein content but normal electrolyte content. There is increased capillary pressure in cardiogenic edema; therefore, reduction of intravascular volume by the use of diuretics or enhancement of venous compliance by the use of vasodilators such as morphine or nitrites will reduce the edema. Resolution of cardiogenic edema is fast with pharmacologic therapy. Since the pulmonary vascular endothelium is essentially undamaged, pulmonary edema clears rapidly once the pulmonary hydrostatic pressure is reduced.

101. The answer is C. *(Neurotransmission and pain)* Endorphins and enkephalins are important opioid-like proteins found in many tissues, including the central nervous system (CNS). The central origin of each peptide is confirmed by their persistence in the brain even after hypophysectomy. Endorphins, but not enkephalins, are synthesized within the anterior pituitary of man from the glycoprotein precursor, pro-opiomelanocortin. There are multiple opioid receptors, and the above peptides are ligands for many of these. Enkephalins, as opposed to endorphins, appear to be active in suppressing afferent sensory pain input in the spinal cord by affecting substance P–containing nerve endings. Both opioids are capable of producing states of analgesia, sedation, and respiratory depression via central actions.

102. The answer is C. *(Antimicrobials)* Cephalosporins are usually sensitive to β-lactamase, which makes many gonococci resistant to penicillin G. Ceftriaxone has proven to be unaffected by β-lactamase and, thus, has become the drug of first choice. Ceftriaxone is a third-generation cephalosporin that is bactericidal by interfering with peptidoglycan synthesis of a number of microbes, thereby affecting their cell wall function. The drug is considerably more expensive than penicillin G, although a single intramuscular dose is usually effective in treating gonorrhea. Like penicillin G, the most serious adverse effect is a hypersensitivity reaction.

103. The answer is D. *(Reverse transcriptase)* Reverse transcriptase is a unique polymerase capable of synthesizing a DNA molecule complementary to an RNA template (e.g., a retrovirus genome). However, the same enzyme can digest the RNA strand (its RNase H activity) and synthesize a DNA molecule complementary to the newly made DNA strand. Thus, it acts as a RNA-dependent DNA polymerase and a DNA-dependent polymerase. It plays a role in the replication of retroviruses and hepadnaviruses (e.g., hepatitis B virus). Reverse transcriptase is a protein not a nucleic acid (genome). Retroviruses are the only RNA viruses that encode such an enzyme.

104. The answer is C. *(Asthma therapy)* Cromolyn sodium inhibits degranulation of mast cells and, in other, poorly understood, ways, interferes with the inflammatory process now assumed to be critical to moderate asthma due to a variety of allergens and other conditions. Cromolyn is not absorbed from the gut and must be administered topically to the lung where it acts prophylactically to inhibit bronchospasm due to inhaled allergens, exercise, or altered environmental conditions. It does not directly relax bronchial smooth muscle in vivo or in vitro and, thus, is of little use in acute emergencies of bronchial hyperreactivity. However, prophylactically, it will reduce the bronchial response to a number of spasmogens.

105. The answer is C. *(Arteries in the axillary region)* The dorsal scapular artery arises from the transverse cervical branch of the thyrocervical artery (trunk), which is a direct branch of the subclavian artery. The subscapular artery and both humeral circumflex arteries are branches of the lower (distal) part of the axillary artery. The supreme thoracic artery arises from the proximal portion of the axillary artery. The axillary artery becomes the brachial artery at the distal margin of the teres major muscle.

106. The answer is D. *(Atherosclerotic involvement of coronary arteries)* The correct order of artery involvement in atherosclerosis from most to least frequent is left anterior descending coronary artery (40% to 50%), right coronary artery (30% to 40%), and left circumflex coronary artery (15% to 20%).

107 and 108. The answers are: 107-C, 108-C. *(Vitamin K deficiency)* A prolonged period of malnutrition and broad-spectrum antibiotics is a common combination that frequently results in vitamin K deficiency. The possibility of an acquired inhibitor was excluded by the mixing test, the patient has not been massively transfused, and folate deficiency is not associated with abnormalities of the coagulation cascade. Von Willebrand's disease does not affect the prothrombin time (PT).

Replenishment of vitamin K is simple, without significant adverse effects, and usually results in normalization of the PT within 12 to 24 hours. Although the patient is not bleeding, he is at an increased risk, so treatment is justified. Fresh frozen plasma and cryoprecipitate, however, carry significant risks, and cryoprecipitate does not concentrate the necessary factors. A decision to discontinue the antibiotics must be made on the grounds of the patient's infection, and it would do little acutely to alter the established deficiency.

109. The answer is C. *(Replication cycle of viruses)* During the eclipse phase, infectious virus particles cannot be recovered because the infecting particle has become dissociated and new, progeny particles have not yet been assembled. The end of the eclipse period is signalled by the appearance of the first detectable progeny virus particles either intracellularly or extracellularly. Distractor (B) could be considered correct only for viruses that bud from the cell and not for viruses that accumulate inside the cell before lysis. There is no parallel between the process of mitosis in eukaryotic cells and the steps in virus replication.

110. The answer is E. *(Menstrual cycle)* The levels of follicle-stimulating hormone (FSH) and luteinizing hormone (LH) are low after ovulation, which is indicated in this illustration by the dotted line. Ovulation usually occurs immediately after the surge in LH and FSH. Little is known about the hormonal basis of the surge; however, it appears to be related to the positive feedback of estrogen on the hypothalamopituitary axis. Body temperature rises immediately after ovulation under the influence of progesterone. Although the production of both LH and FSH declines in the postovulatory period, these hormones continue to influence the secretion of estradiol and progesterone by ovarian theca-lutein and granulosa-lutein cells. This causes secretory changes in the endometrium, which are considerably different from the proliferative changes that occur in the preovulatory phase.

111. The answer is A. *(IgE-mediated hypersensitivity)* The scientist has developed an allergy after repeated exposure to the rodent. The late symptom complex was induced by mast cells triggered by previous interaction of rodent antigen with IgE. This is a typical late-phase set of reactions which are mast-cell mediated; no complement is involved. Corticosteroids will block the late reaction. The involvement of histamine is early, not late.

112. The answer is D. *(Renal physiology)* Glucose is actively reabsorbed into the proximal tubules of the kidney by a saturable transport system. At concentrations less than 200 mg/dl, the transport is complete, and there is no glucose in the urine. At concentrations near 300 mg/dl, the transport system is completely saturated and glucose appears in the urine as a function of glomerular filtration. Glomerular filtration rate (GFR) can be calculated from the slope of the filtered curve or the excreted curve after transport has been saturated. The splay in the curve is due to complex interactions of transport kinetics and heterogeneity of nephron function. Nonetheless, the threshold maximal concentration is a useful index of the number of functional nephrons.

113. The answer is E. *(Systemic lupus erythematosus)* Deficiencies of complement factors C1, C4, and C2 are associated with systemic lupus erythematosus (SLE). Anemia (HCT < 34%) is commonly present in SLE as it is often observed in chronic illnesses. Occasionally severe anemia (HCT < 20%) occurs as a hemolytic anemia associated with Coomb's test positivity. Antibodies against single-stranded DNA are observed in several conditions, including SLE, drug-induced SLE, Sjögren's syndrome, and mixed connective tissue disease, but anti–double-stranded DNA antibodies are commonly seen only in SLE. Antihistone antibodies are also seen in drug-induced SLE and rheumatoid arthritis. The Venereal Disease Research Laboratory (VDRL) test is notably positive in both syphilis and SLE. The test detects the presence of anticardiolipin antibodies.

114. The answer is E. *(Peristalsis; gastrointestinal physiology)* Although the gut is well-innervated by the parasympathetic and sympathetic nervous systems, a significant amount of neuronal control is exerted by an intrinsic nervous system. In particular, the myenteric plexus, which lies between the longitudinal and circular smooth muscle of the gastrointestinal tract, plays an overriding role in peristalsis. In subjects with congenital absence of the myenteric plexus, peristalsis is weak and the coordinated movements of peristaltic reflex toward the anus will not occur. Parasympathetic innervation will add to gastrointestinal motility by promoting contraction. Although there are abundant afferent sensory nerve fibers in the gut, they respond to many stimuli and appear to contribute to distention-induced changes at high transluminal pressures.

115. The answer is E. *(Inflammatory bowel disease)* Pseudopolyps are swollen, inflammatory tags of mucosa that are characteristic of ulcerative colitis. In Crohn's disease one may also find sarcoid-like granulomas within the submucosal and subserosal areas. Crypt abscesses are another prominent finding of ulcerative colitis that are almost never observed in Crohn's disease.

116. The answer is C. *(Pathophysiology of helminthes)* *Enterobius vermicularis* is the etiologic agent of pinworm, a common disease of American children, although enterobiasis occurs in all age-groups. Pinworm infection is characterized by pruritus ani, which is associated with migration of the pinworm outside the anal canal at night. Gastrointestinal infection with the hookworm *Necator americanus* typically produces epigastric pain and abdominal peristalsis. Gastrointestinal ascariasis caused by *Ascaris lumbricoides* is characterized by abdominal pain and malabsorption syndrome. *Trichuris trichiuria*, the whipworm, is a common cosmopolitan parasite that causes abdominal pain and diarrhea. *Onchocerca volvulus*, a tissue nematode, is the etiologic agent of an ocular infection that normally does not occur in the United States.

117. The answer is C. *(Contractile properties of muscle)* Contractile properties of muscle can be measured when muscle lifts a weight (afterload) and is allowed to shorten (isotonic contraction). In this case, force is equal to afterload. Conditions, however, can be created in which force develops without shortening (isometric contraction). Important considerations in isometric contraction include an optimal length (sarcomere = 2.2 μM) in which force is maximal (shorter or longer lengths are associated with a decrease in force) and increased force due to an increase in strength of electrical stimulation. The latter phenomenom (recruitment of more muscle fibers to be activated) is a major mechanism by which the motor control system can increase the force of contraction. Increased force due to repetitive stimulation is summation, and if the frequency of electrical stimulation is rapid enough, force will rise smoothly to a maximum (tetanus). Excitation–contraction mechanisms involve a critical role for intracellular Ca^{2+} and relaxation is associated with uptake of Ca^{2+} into the sarcoplasmic reticulum by Ca^{2+}-specific pumps.

118. The answer is D. *(Cell-mediated immunity)* An individual with a significant purified protein derivative (PPD) reaction who has never had antitubercular drugs is likely to have viable *Mycobacterium tuberculosis* in some body organ. Miliary tuberculosis may or may not be accompanied by a reaction to PPD. Calcified focal lesions are a late manifestation of *M. tuberculosis* infection; reaction to PPD can occur much earlier. An individual with deficient cell-mediated immunity would not produce a reaction to PPD since the reaction requires adequate cell-mediated immunity. Progressive chronic lung disease can be due to many causes and is irrelevant to the question.

119. The answer is E. *(Thyroid gland)* The thyroid gland is an encapsulated, bilobular structure that synthesizes and secretes calcitonin and the thyroid hormones triiodothyronine (T_3) and thyroxine (T_4). Iodide is actively transported by a Na^+-K^+-ATPase pump into the follicular cell. Parafollicular cells synthesize and secrete calcitonin in response to elevated blood calcium levels. Follicular cells secrete thyroglobulin and iodine into the follicles. Iodination of thyroglobulin occurs at the apical border of the follicular cell.

120. The answer is B. *(Lipid metabolism)* Very low-density lipoprotein (VLDL) is synthesized by the liver and secreted into the blood where the action of lipoprotein lipase on the luminal walls of the capillaries converts it first to intermediate-density lipoprotein (IDL) and then to low-density lipoprotein (LDL). LDL, which is rich in cholesterol esters, is taken up by receptor-mediated endocytosis. The LDL has a single copy of apoprotein B, which interacts with the LDL receptor on the surface of cells prior to uptake. VLDL transports endogenous triglycerides; chylomicrons transport dietary triglycerides. The apoprotein components of the lipoproteins are synthesized in the intestinal enterocyte and the liver. Chylomicrons and VLDLs are assembled in the intestinal enterocyte and liver, respectively. High-density lipoprotein (HDL) is synthesized and secreted by the liver. It is primarily involved in transporting cholesterol from the periphery to the liver.

121–123. The answers are: 121-D, 122-E, 123-A. *(Pathobiology and therapy of schistosomiasis)* The drug of choice for the treatment of schistosomiasis is praziquantel, which is effective against all species of schistosomes that infect humans and is effective against both the immature and the adult schistosomal forms. The drug is a broad-spectrum agent and has relatively few side effects; it can be administered orally.

The antimalarial agent chloroquine does not inhibit folic acid synthesis. In contrast, sulfonamides reduce microbial growth by competitively inhibiting folic acid biosynthesis. The mechanism of action of chloroquine involves intercalation with double-stranded DNA, thus blocking DNA replication and transcription. Chloroquine is also a weak base, and it is believed that it concentrates in and raises the pH of acidic compartments within the malarial parasites, thus reducing mobility.

Adult schistosomes do not multiply in humans. The females lay eggs, which are usually excreted in human feces and hatch in fresh water. A complicated life cycle ensues: The larvae invade a specific intermediate host snail, and after several weeks are released and swim in search of another host. Schistosomes eventually complete their life cycles in humans. The larvae enter via the skin, and an intense transient itching of the skin is often noticed soon after infection. Migration occurs first to the lungs, and then to the liver and other organs. Unlike most other trematodes, the sexes are separate.

124. The answer is D. *(Immunoglobulin structure and function)* Rabbit antiserum would react with the variable regions of the light μ and κ chains of IgM. Myeloma protein is the product of a single or limited number of B-cell clones and hence would have a particular V:D:J; V:J sequence in DNA. Human myeloma protein would present as antigen to rabbit antigenic sites (epitopes), but all the nonvariable region sites would be shared with pooled human IgM from serum and hence be absorbed out. Only those rabbit antibodies specific for that IgM (i.e., rabbit anti–human-idiotypic antibodies) would be remaining.

125. The answer is E. *(Anatomy of the gastrointestinal tract)* During portal hypertension, dilated and tortuous veins (varices) often form at sites of anastomoses between the portal and systemic circulations. Esophageal varices form where the left gastric vein anastomoses with veins draining into the azygos and hemiazygos systems. Varices also form where veins from the duodenum and spleen anastomose with renal veins. Caput medusae are varices in the abdominal wall that form where periumbilical veins anastomose with superior and inferior epigastric veins. Hemorrhoids are varices that often form in channels between the three rectal veins. Veins from the jejunum drain only into the portal circulation; therefore, no varices develop.

126. The answer is D. *(Hepatitis B incubation)* Hepatitis B has a long incubation period, which may extend as long as 160 days but rarely surpasses that length of time; it rarely is under 45 days. Hepatitis B generally is associated with instruments contaminated by infectious blood or blood products. The route of infection is via direct inoculation of the infectious material into the blood.

127. The answer is B. *(Recurrent urinary tract infections)* The increased adherence of pathogenic bacteria to vaginal epithelial cells is currently the only demonstrable biologic difference that can be shown in women susceptible to urinary tract infections.

128–130. The answers are: 128-C, 129-B, 130-D. *(Pathology of myocardial infarction)* A fast rhythm with a wide complex is usually consistent with a ventricular tachycardia. It is highly likely that the 60-year-old man described in the question suffered a myocardial infarction associated with a ventricular tachycardia (and essentially sudden death). The treatment of choice for ventricular tachycardia associated with myocardial ischemia is lidocaine.

Lidocaine is typical of the group of antiarrhythmic agents that block Na^+ channels, which are the current-carrying processes responsible for depolarization in fast fibers of the heart (ventricular and atrial). It suppresses these channels in the infarct area in cells with abnormal resting membrane potential. Although the mechanism underlying this selectivity is poorly understood, it is thought that perhaps abnormal tissue ion channels tend to be in inactivated states, increasing the binding and efficacy of state-dependent agents, or that damaged myocardial tissue tends to accumulate agents such as lidocaine to a greater degree. Agents such as diltiazem, propranolol, or digitalis affect electrical propagation and conduction in SA and AV nodal tissue where parasympathetic input predominates and Ca^+ is the current-carrying ion. Although propranolol has been shown to have some utility in reducing subsequent damage after myocardial infarction, it is contraindicated in patients with hypotension (and potential poor left ventricular function). Epinephrine increases oxygen demands on the heart by directly stimulating myocardial β-receptors as well as increasing afterload and in this case appears to be contraindicated.

Creatine kinase (CK) is an enzyme that catalyzes the transfer of high-energy phosphates and is found largely in tissues that use large amounts of energy. The two common isoforms are CK-MM (muscle) and CK-BB (brain). There is an isoform that contains both M and B subunits (CK-MB), which is found only in the myocardium. In the heart, CK is approximately 85% CK-MM and 15% CK-MB. An increase in both total CK and CK-MB (secondary to myocardial injury) has proven to be highly sensitive and specific in the diagnosis of myocardial infarction. Lactate dehydrogenase (LDH) is often elevated 48 to 72 hours after injury, and it is usually the LDH_1 isoenzyme (myocardial-associated) rather than LDH_5 (skeletal muscle and liver) that is used for the diagnosis of myocardial injury. Aspartate aminotransferase levels increase after myocardial infarction, and, in general, are of little value in light of the above noted changes in CK (and LDH) isoenzymes.

Significant injury to the anterior wall of the left ventricle may be due to occlusion (>70%) of the left anterior descending coronary artery. Alternatively, occlusion to a lesser degree of the left mainstem coronary artery may also produce the above pathology. The left circumflex artery may affect the anterior wall but is more likely to involve inferior posterior parts of the heart.

131. The answer is B. *(Extracellular matrix production and chondroblasts)* Chondroblasts are cartilage cells located deep in the perichondrium, the dense connective capsule that surrounds cartilage. As chondroblasts secrete extracellular matrix rich in type II collagen and cartilage proteoglycan, they become surrounded by their own extracellular matrix and differentiate into chondrocytes. Both chondroblasts and chondrocytes are capable of cell division by mitosis. The endosteum is a layer of osteoblasts in bone. The periosteum is the outer connective tissue covering of bone.

132. The answer is B. *(Anticoagulants)* Heparin is a large, water-soluble polymer that must be given parenterally and does not cross the placenta. It is primarily used for acute anticoagulant therapy because its onset of action is rapid. It can be reversed by the administration of protamine. The main action of heparin is thought to involve catalyzing the activation of antithrombin III in blood, thereby inhibiting thrombin and factor Xa. Warfarin affects normal synthesis of clotting factors in the liver and its anticoagulant effects can be reversed by vitamin K. It is well-absorbed orally but will cross the placenta and may affect the fetus. It is used on a chronic basis for deep venous thrombosis and long-term care post–myocardial infarction because it is slow in onset of action.

133. The answer is A. *(Cholesterol biosynthesis)* Lovastatin is a natural product that inhibits 3-hydroxy-3-methylglutaryl coenzyme A (HMG CoA) in the liver and, in a complicated fashion, causes an increase in high-affinity low-density lipoprotein (LDL) receptors. Accordingly, it is receiving extensive use in people with familial hyperlipidemias and hypercholesterolemias with elevated LDLs. Other lipid-lowering drugs have distinctly different actions, including reduced hepatic secretion of very low-density lipoprotein (VLDL) [niacin], binding of bile acids in the intestine (cholestyramine), enhanced clearance of triglyceride-rich lipoproteins (clofibrate), and poorly understood mechanisms that can have the adverse effect of reducing high-density lipoproteins (HDL) [probucol].

134. The answer is B. *(Epidermis)* The order of epidermal maturation is stratum basale, stratum spinosum, stratum granulosum, stratum lucidum, and stratum corneum. The stratum basale is the germinal layer of the epidermis. Cells migrate and differentiate from this layer at a rate equal to desquamation of keratin from the outermost layer. The stratum spinosum is superficial to the stratum basale, and its cells are in the process of growth and early keratin synthesis. The stratum granulosum is characterized by the presence of intracellular granules, which contribute to the keratinization process. The stratum lucidum is a homogeneous layer between the stratum granulosum and the stratum corneum that is present only in thick skin. The stratum corneum is the most superficial layer of the epidermis and is mainly composed of keratin.

135. The answer is D. *(Cranial sinuses)* The cavernous sinus drains into the superior and inferior petrosal sinuses. The great vein of Galen joins with the inferior sagittal sinus to form the straight sinus, which joins the superior sagittal and occipital sinuses to form the confluence of sinuses. The left and right transverse sinuses drain from the confluence and become the sigmoid sinus, which joins the internal jugular vein inferior to the skull.

136. The answer is D. *(Immune response; secondary exposure)* The preferred treatment method for this woman is tetanus toxoid because it will stimulate her anamnestic active response. Equine tetanus globulin would passively immunize the patient to tetanus but could cause immediate or subsequent serum sickness. Administration of human tetanus immune globulin would result in passive immunity. *Clostridium tetani* is not sensitive to aminoglycosides.

137. The answer is A. *(Neuroendocrinology and pituitary function)* Prolactin synthesis from the anterior pituitary is under basal regulation by several inhibiting factors, including dopamine. Therefore, bromocriptine has the predicted effect of decreasing prolactin synthesis in normal subjects. In women at parturition, this will result in inhibition of lactation without pain or engorgement of the breast. In women with pituitary tumors that cause infertility problems due to hyperprolactinemia, bromocriptine has been useful in reversing the galactorrhea and amenorrhea and, thus, restoring reproductive potential. Bromocriptine is paradoxically useful in patients with acromegaly by inhibiting growth hormone. In contrast to normal subjects in which dopamine promotes growth hormone release, in acromegaly there is a presumptive expansion of stem cells (e.g., somatomammotrophs). Dopaminergic agents are limited in usefulness because of significant side effects, including nausea.

138. The answer is D. *(Epithelia)* Stratified squamous epithelium lines the mouth, pharynx, esophagus, vagina, and anal canal. It also comprises the epidermis. Stratified squamous epithelium consists of several layers of cells with a superficial layer of flattened, anucleated cells. It may be keratinized or nonkeratinized. In contrast, simple squamous epithelium is a single layer of flattened, nonkeratinized cells, which lines the pleural, pericardial, and peritoneal cavities.

139. The answer is C. *(Hematocele)* Hematocele is the accumulation of blood in the tunica vaginalis. It usually occurs after trauma to the testis, but it may be associated with torsion of the testis, widespread hemorrhagic disease, or an invasive tumor.

140. The answer is B. *(Renal clearance)* Clearance is the theoretical volume of plasma cleaned (or cleared) per unit time and in the kidney may be calculated by the ratio of the amount excreted ($U_x \cdot \dot{V}$) and P_x. Solution of this equation with the given data yields a calculated clearance of 125 ml/min, which is identical to the glomerular filtration rate (GFR) [renal blood flow $\times$ glomerular filtration fraction, or 500×0.25]. Thus, substance x is neither secreted nor reabsorbed and is a useful indicator of the glomerular filtration, such as inulin. Frequently, endogenous creatinine clearance is used as a quantitative measure of the GFR. Creatinine is a useful estimate since it is largely cleared by filtration. However, values are higher than inulin values because there is a slight amount of tubular secretion of creatinine.

141. The answer is B. *(Median nerve)* The median nerve supplies most of the extrinsic flexor muscles of the hand, including the flexor pollicis longus, the flexor digitorum superficialis, and the radial half of the flexor digitorum profundus. It also supplies muscles of the thenar compartment, including the opponens pollicis, the abductor pollicis brevis, and the superficial head of the flexor pollicis brevis, which flex the thumb. Median nerve palsy affects all of these muscles; therefore, a patient with median nerve palsy is not able to oppose the thumb or flex digits two and three and exhibits thenar atrophy. A claw hand deformity, in which paralyzed digits are semiflexed by an intact flexor digitorum superficialis, is caused by an ulnar lesion and is not present in median nerve palsy.

142. The answer is D. *(Alzheimer's disease)* Lewy bodies are characteristic of idiopathic Parkinson's disease, not Alzheimer's disease. Clinical characteristics of Alzheimer's disease include progressive disorientation, memory loss, and aphasia. Major microscopic features include neurofibrillary tangles, neuritic (senile) plaques, amyloid angiopathy, granulovacuolar degeneration, and Hirano bodies.

143. The answer is A. *(Antigen–antibody interaction)* HSA and DNP-BGG are not precipitated by the same antibodies; therefore, there are no overlapping spurs or line of identity. Anti-DNP antibodies react with DNP hapten on DNP-BGG, DNP-BSA, and DNP-HSA. BSA and HSA share some determinants seen by the polyclonal antibody, which sees more determinants on BSA (the immunogen) than on HSA. Anti-BSA antibodies detect no determinants on BGG and, therefore, do not form a precipitin line.

144. The answer is D. *(Myeloid metaplasia)* Bone marrow hypocellularity and teardrop-shaped erythrocytes are pathognomonic for myeloid metaplasia with myelofibrosis. Leukocyte alkaline phosphatase levels are normal or elevated until the final stages of the disease. The liver does not usually undergo any significant change in size, whereas the spleen is almost always markedly enlarged as it becomes the principal site of extramedullary hematopoiesis.

145. The answer is B. *(Antibody production)* During the course of a viral infection, the patient's specific antibody will rise. Differences in the titers of antibodies must differ by greater than twofold in order to be significant. In the data presented, the concentration of echovirus type 4 antibodies rose eightfold compared to twofold differences in the other antibodies tested. Thus, the patient experienced an infection caused by echovirus type 4.

146. The answer is D. *(Cardiac cycle)* The T wave or loop is caused by ventricular repolarization. Although the wave is due to repolarization, it is opposite the zero reference line from the P wave, which is caused by atrial depolarization. The portion of ventricular muscle that repolarizes first is the large portion covering the entire outer surface of the ventricles; the endocardial areas repolarize last. Repolarization is slowest in the endocardium due to compression of myocardial capillaries during ventricular contraction. Thus, the predominant direction of the vector through the heart during ventricular repolarization is from base to apex, which is similar to the vector during depolarization of the ventricle.

147. The answer is C. *(Human genetics and isohemagglutinin titers)* The Rh type of the child could not be definitively determined from the test. Anti-B antisera react with the child's red blood cells. The child's serum reacts with A+ red blood cells, and, therefore, the child is BB or BO. It is possible that the child is the natural offspring, so distractors (A), (B), and (D) are not valid.

148. The answer is A. *(Intercostal nerves)* Intercostal nerves are the anterior rami of the first 11 thoracic spinal nerves; the 12th thoracic nerve gives rise to the subcostal nerve.

149. The answer is C. *(Age-related immunological changes)* The patient developed a ragweed allergy by losing the specific T8+ suppressor cells that held his B cells or their specific helpers in check. Thymus function decreases with age.

150. The answer is E. *(Muscle physiology)* Visceral smooth muscle is considerably smaller than skeletal muscle and requires less energy to sustain the same tension of contraction. Visceral smooth muscle is similar to skeletal muscle in that it has actin and myosin and can respond to various stimuli by initiating an action potential. However, entry of Ca^{2+} via slowly opening Ca^{2+} channels is both responsible for the action potential as well as for interacting with actin and myosin contractile elements to cause contraction.

151. The answer is C. *(Coronary arteries)* An infarct that includes the atrioventricular (AV) node probably is caused by an occluded right coronary artery. The AV node is located in the lower part of the atrial septum, just above the attachment of the septal cusp of the tricuspid valve. This area, the right ventricle, and the interventricular septum are supplied by the posterior descending (interventricular) branch of the right coronary artery in 85% to 90% of people.

152. The answer is C. *(Respiratory gas exchange)*

$$P_{ACO_2} = (\dot{V}_{CO_2})k/\dot{V}_A$$

where k is a constant and $\dot{V}_{CO_2}$ is carbon dioxide production and $\dot{V}_A$ is alveolar ventilation. Thus, doubling $\dot{V}_A$ will decrease alveolar (and thus arterial) P_{CO_2} by half. Alveolar P_{O_2} will have a tendency to increase since

$$P_{AO_2} = (P_B - P_{H_2O})(F_{IO_2}) - (P_{ACO_2})(k)$$

where P_B is barometric pressure, P_{H_2O} is water vapor pressure and F_{IO_2} is the fraction of inspired air that is oxygen.

153. The answer is D. *(Hormone replacement therapy)* Intermittent therapy with gonadotropin-releasing hormone (Gn-RH) is useful as a mimic of normal hypothalamic function and causes increased synthesis of both follicle-stimulating hormone (FSH) and luteinizing hormone (LH). This may be useful in restoring a normal menstrual cycle in some women with hypothalamic pituitary disorders. In contrast, constant infusion of high doses of Gn-RH decreases gonadotropin release. This application may be useful as a novel and specific contraceptive therapy as well as useful hormonal therapy for some prostate cancers.

154. The answer is E. *(Autonomic pharmacology)* A drug which might worsen the symptoms of myasthenia gravis is d-tubocurarine. Although the reasons for the development of the autoimmune basis of myasthenia gravis remain obscure, the overall effect is a reduction in effective receptors at the neuromuscular junction. Neurotransmitter release is normal, but the amplitude of the end-plate potential is greatly reduced, which increases the likelihood of failure of neurotransmission. Agents, such as neostigmine (anticholinesterase drugs), that increase the half-life of released acetylcholine are of significant therapeutic benefit. Patients with myasthenia gravis are supersensitive to nondepolarizing muscle relaxants, such as d-tubocurarine, because the margin of safety of the drugs is reduced.

155. The answer is A. *(Neurotransmitter reuptake)* A significant effect of imipramine is its ability to inhibit neuronal re-uptake of norepinephrine by blocking the presynaptic carrier site for this process. Therefore, imipramine would be expected to interfere with antihypertensive agents that require this uptake mechanism. The hypotensive effects of methyldopa (a commonly used antihypertensive agent) depend upon this amine being taken up into neuronal presynaptic sites and subsequently being decarboxylated and hydroxylated to the false neurotransmitter α-methylnoradrenaline. α-Methylnorepinephrine is weaker than norepinephrine for α_1 stimulation and is a potent α_2-adrenergic agonist, causing increased presynaptic inhibition of norepinephrine release in peripheral nerve terminals and, perhaps more importantly, having a potent α_2-mediated central effect that reduces sympathetic outflow from the central nervous system (CNS). Thus, imipramine tends to impair the effect of methyldopa.

156. The answer is D. *(Transplantation and MHC matching)* An AB host will be tolerant of both A and B cells, but immunocompetent spleen cells of strain BB will recognize A determinants on a host and mount an immune response. Distractor (A) is a complete match. In distractor (B), immunocompetent AB bone marrow cells see the BB host as self. In distractor (C), graft cells are not immunocompetent.

157. The answer is D. *(Etiology and diagnosis of urinary tract infections)* *Escherichia coli* is the most common etiologic agent of simple urinary tract infection (UTI) in unhospitalized ambulatory people who are otherwise healthy. This member of the Enterobacteriaceae family accounts for about 50% of UTIs in these people. *Klebsiella pneumoniae* is the second most common cause of UTI in this population, accounting for 8% to 13% of disease. *Staphylococcus aureus* is only an occasional cause of UTI; *Serratia marcescens* is a common cause of UTI in hospitalized and debilitated patients with indwelling urinary catheters. *Gardnerella vaginalis* is an occasional etiologic agent of vulvovaginitis.

158–161. The answers are: 158-B, 159-E, 160-B, 161-A. *(Cell biology)* Proteins are synthesized by large ribonucleoprotein complexes called ribosomes using mRNA as a template. Proteins destined for transport to the Golgi apparatus, the lysosomes, the plasma membrane, or the exterior of the cell are synthesized in association with the endoplasmic reticulum. Growth factor receptors are plasma membrane proteins, which can be internalized by receptor-mediated endocytosis. Glycosylation is one of the major biosynthetic functions of the endoplasmic reticulum, which occurs first as the protein is passing into the lumen of this organelle. This initial glycosylation is followed by several processing steps, one of which is the addition of terminal sialic acids in the Golgi apparatus.

162. The answer is E. *(Etiology of bacterial endocarditis)* The viridans streptococci account for more than 50% of all cases of bacterial endocarditis. *Staphylococcus aureus* and *Staphylococcus epidermidis* are important causes of acute and subacute endocarditis, respectively, especially following thoracic surgery. Anaerobic gram-positive cocci, such as *Peptococcus* species, rarely have been associated with endocarditis. Strongyloides and necator are intestinal roundworms, not bacteria.

163. The answer is A. *(Erythroblastosis fetalis)* In a subsequent pregnancy, the woman's fetus could be B, Rh$^+$. If so, the B, Rh$^+$ fetus could develop erythroblastosis fetalis. Anti-Rb antibodies are often IgG and can pass from the mother to the Rh$^+$ fetus. All immunocompetent B individuals have anti-A antibodies elicited by bacterial flora. If a subsequent fetus is Rh$^-$, it cannot develop erythroblastosis fetalis because the disease is caused by the anti-Rh$^+$ antibodies reacting with Rh$^+$ fetal blood cells. Distractor (D) is false because anti-Rh antibodies do not "naturally" occur.

164. The answer is D. *(Autonomic pharmacology)* Atropine is a relatively lipid-soluble compound that has both central and peripheral antimuscarinic effects. It is often used to increase heart rate by virtue of its vagolytic effects. It is widely used as an adjunct in surgical premedication because it aids in maintaining airway patency by dilating bronchial smooth muscle and inhibiting airway secretions. Urinary retention is one of the few clinical conditions in which a muscarinic agonist, such as bethanechol, is used therapeutically.

165. The answer is C. *(Regulation of respiration)* Although CO_2 will stimulate carotid chemoreceptors and increase ventilation, this effect is small (especially with normal P_{O_2} and pH) compared to its stimulation of central chemoreceptors located in the ventral surface of the medulla oblongata. CO_2 is generally thought to convert to H^+ and HCO_3^- in the cerebrospinal fluid (CSF) and extracellular space of the ventral surface of the medulla oblongata. The H^+ subsequently stimulates chemoreceptors in the region, which increases respiratory activity. J fibers in the lung respond to mechanical stimuli, including interstitial water changes.

166. The answer is D. *(Principles of combination chemotherapy)* Combinations of anticancer agents are often used to increase the tumoricidal activity of each agent. Combinations are often cytotoxic to heterogeneous populations of cancer cells and can be arranged to affect both dividing and resting cells. The agents should have different mechanisms of action as well as different toxic side effects. Cross-resistance between the agents should be avoided.

167. The answer is B. *(Characteristics of African trypanosomiasis and malaria)* African trypanosomiasis and malaria both present initially with periodic febrile attacks. The endemic areas for both diseases overlap in sub-Saharan Africa. Malaria is characterized by fever, anemia, and splenomegaly. Sporozoa of the genus *Plasmodium* infect erythrocytes and hepatic parenchymal cells. The parasites are carried by female *Anopheles* mosquitoes.

African trypanosomiasis (sleeping sickness) is caused by *Trypanosoma brucei* infection, which is transmitted by blood-sucking tsetse flies. *T. brucei* adopts behavior to avoid the immune response of the host. Trypanosomes enter the bloodstream through lymphatics and undergo extracellular division in the bloodstream, cerebrospinal fluid, and interstitial spaces. This involves the organism altering its external antigens every 5 to 6 days; therefore, the parasitemia occurs in cycles, and each cycle of infection is antigenically different.

168. The answer is D. *(Congestive heart failure therapy)* Digitalis inhibits the Na^+-K^+ ATPase of the cell membrane, thereby inhibiting the Na^+-K^+ pump. This effect is enhanced during conditions of hypokalemia, presumably because there is less competition to the common K^+–binding site. Inhibition of the pump leads to an increase in intracellular Na^+, which decreases Ca^{2+} extrusion via the Na^+-Ca^{2+} exchange. Accordingly, intracellular Ca^{2+} concentrations are elevated, accounting for the positive inotropic effect of digitalis. Digitalis has significant indirect effects, including an increase in vagal tone that affects cardiac electrical activity. The therapeutic index for digitalis is extraordinarily low for an agent that is so commonly used and has led to a careful dosing regimen with considerable attention to biologic and chemical indicators of digitalis toxicity.

169. The answer is C. *(Muscles of the leg)* Muscles passing anterior to the transverse axis of the ankle dorsiflex the foot. The tendon of the peroneus brevis muscle passes posterior to the transverse axis and thus aids in plantar flexion.

170. The answer is A. *(Hypersensitivity reactions)* Complement activation is not normally seen in type I hypersensitivity immune reactions. Hives (urticaria) are commonly seen in type I IgE-mediated hypersensitivity immune responses. Mast cell degranulation within the lesion releases histamine and a slow-reacting substance of anaphylaxis, along with other materials. Aspirin use is contraindicated because it inhibits the production of prostaglandins, which tend to retard IgE-dependent mast cell degranulation, not because of the age of the child.

171. The answer is D. *(Hyperthyroidism therapy)* Propylthiouracil (PTU) and similar agents (methimazole) are well-absorbed after oral administration. They are used for the treatment of hyperthyroidism and, occasionally, are the sole agents used (especially in children) until remission occurs. These agents inhibit thyroperoxidase-catalyzed oxidation and peripheral deiodination of T_4 to T_3. They usually take several weeks to return abnormal conditions, such as elevated basal metabolism, to control values in patients with Graves' disease. There is concern regarding fetal effects of these agents since they do cross the placenta and enter breast milk; thus, the issue of iatrogenic cretinism needs to be considered.

172. The answer is A. *(Nonsteroidal anti-inflammatory agents and gout therapy)* Acetaminophen has very little anti-inflammatory effect and is not predicted to be useful in gout. Agents used in the treatment of gout may act to affect the metabolic disposition of uric acid crystals or interfere with the inflammatory process that accompanies this genetically determined disorder. Thus, allopurinol inhibits xanthine oxidase and reduces uric acid synthesis. Sulfinpyrazone increases uric acid secretion by the renal tubules. Colchicine binds to tubulin and interferes with the motility of neutrophils that may contribute to the attack. Acetylsalicylic acid (aspirin) has an overall anti-inflammatory effect that is also useful.

173. The answer is C. *(Oxidative phosphorylation)* An uncoupler will inhibit oxygen consumption. The chemosmotic theory of oxidative phosphorylation is based on the tenet that the energy-linked phosphorylation of adenosine diphosphate (ADP) is driven by a proton gradient across the inner mitochondrial membrane. Due to the tight coupling of oxidation and phosphorylation, agents that block electron transport will also inhibit phosphorylation. Similarly, agents that inhibit adenosine triphosphate (ATP) synthesis will reduce the rate of electron transport. Uncouplers of oxidative phosphorylation are compounds that allow mitochondria to use oxygen even though ATP synthesis may not be occurring. Substrates oxidized in reactions producing reduced nicotinamide adenine dinucleotide (NADH) have P:O ratios of 3; substrates that are flavin adenine dinucleotide (FAD)-linked have a P:O ratio of 2. Electrons from $FADH_2$ enter the electron transport chain distal to complex I, which provides the energy for the synthesis of one ATP molecule.

174. The answer is C. *(Retroviruses)* Human immunodeficiency virus (HIV) is a replication-competent retrovirus because it contains all of the genes necessary for its replication. Acute-transforming viruses, which exist among the avian and murine retroviruses, are defined as retroviruses possessing defective genomes (i.e., they have lost crucial virus genes in exchange for cellular gene sequences that can act as oncogenes). An endogenous virus is one whose genetic information is carried by every cell in a given animal species and is thus vertically transmitted via the egg and sperm. HIV is transmitted horizontally as an infectious disease; it is not present in the cells of uninfected individuals. Oncoviruses comprise a group of retroviruses distinct from the lentiviruses.

175–180. The answers are: 175-E, 176-A, 177-D, 178-C, 179-C, 180-B. *(Pathophysiology and treatment of gout)* Of the tests listed in the question, synovial fluid analysis, erythrocyte sedimentation rate, C-reactive protein, and differential white blood cell count may be useful in discriminating inflammatory versus noninflammatory musculoskeletal disorders. Synovial fluid analysis reveals clear liquid containing long, needle-shaped, negatively birefringent intracellular crystals (sodium urate). The presence of these crystals and their ingestion by macrophages are typical findings with gout.

Neurologic workup reveals slight dysarthria and incoordination. These symptoms are sequelae of an inherited X-linked partial deficiency of hypoxanthine–guanine phosphoribosyltransferase. This enzyme converts hypoxanthine to inosinic acid. Its deficiency elevates purine synthesis, which contributes to the hyperuricemia of gout. Lesch-Nyhan victims are identifiable at birth and are mentally retarded. Osteoarthritis and calcium hydroxyapatite deposition disease afflict the elderly.

Colchicine is the anti-inflammatory drug of choice for gout. Allopurinol inhibits xanthine oxidase, the enzyme that converts hypoxanthine to xanthine, and xanthine to uric acid. Thus, allopurinol decreases urate production and is efficacious for the treatment of gout.

181. The answer is B. *(Congenital heart disease)* Tetralogy of Fallot, a common cause of neonatal cyanosis, is a combination of four abnormalities: pulmonary valve stenosis, ventricular septal defect, aorta overriding the septal defect, and right ventricular hypertrophy. This syndrome does not involve a patent ductus arteriosus.

182. The answer is E. *(Coenzymes)* Coenzymes are carriers in many biochemical reactions. Many water-soluble vitamins, which serve as precursors for coenzymes, have adenine nucleotides as a part of their structure. Reduced nicotinamide-adenine dinucleotide (NADH) and reduced nicotinamide-adenine dinucleotide phosphate (NADPH) are carriers of a hydride ion in oxidation–reduction reactions. Pyridoxal phosphate is a carrier of amino groups in many reactions involving amino acids. Thiamine pyrophosphate is important in carbohydrate metabolism as a carrier of aldehyde groups. Biotin is a carrier of carboxyl groups and becomes covalently attached to a number of carboxylases.

183. The answer is B. *(Life cycle of herpesvirus)* Herpesviruses are notorious for remaining latent in neurons of sensory ganglia, where upon activation they can replicate and cause a variety of diseases. Once activated, epithelial cells may become infected, but upon subsidence of disease, herpesvirus components are not found in these cells. Autoimmune diseases are not caused by herpesviruses. Herpesvirus replication takes place in the nucleus of infected cells.

184. The answer is A. *(Berry aneurysms)* There is no known association between chronic hypertension and the development or rupture of berry aneurysms. Berry aneurysms are not present at birth, and they form most often at the bifurcation of cerebral arteries. A discontinuity of smooth muscle in the arterial wall causes it to bulge outward; rupture may occur due to acute rise in intravascular pressure. Approximately 10% to 30% of patients with adult (autosomal dominant) polycystic kidney disease develop berry aneurysms, which occur most commonly in the circle of Willis.

185. The answer is C. *(Edema)* Edema occurs in cirrhosis of the liver, congestive heart failure, kwashiorkor, and nephrotic syndrome but not in systemic hypertension. Edema is the abnormal expansion of the interstitial fluid or the accumulation of fluid in an extracellular space, such as the peritoneal cavity. It results from increased hydrostatic pressure in the venous system, decreased oncotic pressure, sodium retention, or lymphatic destruction. In contrast, edema does not occur in systemic hypertension because arterial vessels are relatively impermeable.

186 and 187. The answers are: 186-B, 187-D. *(Androgen actions and autonomic control of bladder)* The prostate depends upon androgens for its structural and functional activity. Dihydrotestosterone — the metabolically active androgen in prostate cells — is converted from testosterone by α-reductase in the cytoplasm. Phenylpropanolamine is an α-sympathomimetic, which can tighten the periurethral smooth muscle of the bladder neck and increase bladder neck outlet resistance.

188. The answer is B. *(Nissl substance)* Nissl substance does not contain DNA, lipid, glycogen, or synaptic vesicles. Nissl substance is basophilic because it contains ribosomes, which are bound to endoplasmic reticulum or are free in the cytoplasm. Basic dyes interact with anionic groups. In Nissl substance, the anionic groups are the phosphate groups of RNA (ribosomes).

189. The answer is A. *(Lysozyme production and paneth cells)* Paneth cells secrete lysozyme, an antibacterial enzyme, and are found in the crypts of Lieberkuhn in the small intestine. Pepsinogen is secreted by chief cells in the lower half of the fundic glands. Intrinsic factor and hydrochloric acid are secreted by parietal (oxyntic) cells in gastric glands. Gastrin is secreted by G cells [which are a specific type of amine precursor uptake and decarboxylation (APUD) cells].

190. The answer is A. *(Coagulative necrosis)* Coagulative necrosis, the most common form of necrosis, occurs most often after acute severe ischemia in organs such as the heart, kidney, or adrenal gland. Characteristically, the basic cellular shape is preserved; however, the nuclei disappear, and the cytoplasm is coagulated, granular, and acidophilic. Infiltration of leukocytes removes necrotic cells by proteolytic degradation and phagocytosis.

191. The answer is E. *(Gastric secretion)* Concentrating H^+ into gastric secretion is a poorly understood active process associated with parietal cells. Most current theories have suggested that active transport of chloride (Cl^-) from cytoplasm to lumen causes an electrogenic gradient for the translocation of K^+. At the luminal surface, H^+ is actively secreted into the canaliculus of the parietal cell in exchange for K^+ via H^+-K^+ ATPase. Carbon dioxide formed within the cell or from blood combines with water and is hydrolyzed to carbonic acid (HCO_3^-). HCO_3^- dissociates, and the excretion of bicarbonate (H_2CO_3) in exchange for Cl^- contributes to the overall movement of H^+ to the lumen. Inhibition of the formation of HCO_3^- with acetazolamide, a carbonic acid anhydrase inhibitor, will virtually stop the secretion of H^+. Increases in H^+ secretion are associated with increased vagal tone (acetylcholine as neurotransmitter) or local production of histamine. These neurohumoral inputs contribute to the pharmacologic strategies of depressing H^+ secretion in ulcerative disorders with anticholinergics and antihistamines, respectively. The presence of food, either directly or by the release of secretagogues, causes the delivery of gastrin to the parietal cells. Gastrin is an important polypeptide that increases H^+ secretion.

192. The answer is C. *(Mycobacterium tuberculosis)* *Mycobacterium tuberculosis* is transmitted only by infected humans, whereas *Mycobacterium avium-intracellulare* is a soil mycobacterium that is not contagious. Furthermore, *M. tuberculosis* does require treatment, and the patient should be treated to prevent spread.

193. The answer is D. *(Infection and immunity; phagocytosis)* An assay for the myeloperoxidase activity of neutrophils would indicate that the neutrophils were capable of killing phagocytized bacteria. Basophils, T cells (CD4 or CD8), and anti-tetanus and diphtheria antibodies are not crucial in fighting off staphylococcus infections. They provide some information about the immune status of the patient but cannot indicate if the neutrophils, the primary phagocytic cell in this kind of infection, are functioning in the patient.

194–204. The answers are: 194-B, 195-B, 196-C, 197-A, 198-D, 199-C, 200-C, 201-B, 202-C, 203-A, 204-C. *(Infectious diseases)* Sergeant Able most likely has been infected by enterotoxic *Escherichia coli*. *Shigella dysenteria*, *Campylobacter jejuni*, and *Entamoeba histolytica* usually cause more pronounced disease, and, because they are invasive, infection results in blood and leukocytes in the stool. Malaria (infection by *Plasmodium falciparum*) causes fever and chills; therefore it is not under consideration. *E. coli* enteritis is classically acquired by eating unsanitary food. Enteric disease is not transmitted by mosquitoes. Ready-to-eat meals (REMs), alcoholic beverages, and hot tea are basically sterile. Sergeant Able's symptoms do not warrant aggressive treatment, although rehydration and control of the diarrhea are necessary.

Sergeant Baker's symptoms are unmistakably those of shigellosis. Blood and leukocytes in the stools rule out staphylococcal food poisoning; amebiasis is much more indolent in its initial stages than Sergeant Baker's infection; the initial symptoms of typhoid (i.e., extreme weakness, anorexia, and drowsiness as well as diarrhea) are not the symptoms in this case; and cholera is not considered because of the indications of invasiveness. Rehydration and antibiotic therapy are recommended. Loperamide is contraindicated when blood and leukocytes are present in the stool.

The Iraqi officer has unmistakable symptoms of cholera, particularly the rice-water stool and motile bacteria. *Vibrio cholerae* should be cultured in an alkaline medium. The organism is slightly basophilic and can readily be enriched in an alkaline peptone broth (pH 8.4), which suppresses the growth of other intestinal microorganisms. Intravenous rehydration is the gold standard of cholera treatment; it is life-saving. Tetracycline will reduce the duration of the illness.

The time sequence of Lieutenant Doug's symptoms and his disturbed mentation argue strongly for typhoid fever, caused by *Salmonella typhi*. Laboratory diagnosis would indicate the presence of *S. typhi* in blood, urine, and stool at various stages of the illness. Typhoid is a typical water-borne disease, and coffee could not harbor viable organisms since it is usually served hot. REMs presumably are devoid of pathogens. There is no record of *S. typhi* transmission via sexual intercourse.

205. The answer is B. *(Chagas disease)* Patients with chronic Chagas disease present with cardiac conduction defects. The other signs and symptoms listed are classic for several diseases that are endemic in Central and South America, including malaria, visceral and cutaneous leishmaniasis, and amebiasis. Chronic Chagas disease (chronic trypanosomiasis) results from gradual tissue destruction of the heart, most likely due to damage to myofibrils and the autonomic innervation of the heart. This results in the conduction defects and megacardia that are hallmarks of the disease. Parasitemia at this point is subpatent; parasites are difficult to detect in either the blood or tissues. Periodic fever and chills are indicative of malaria. Cutaneous and mucocutaneous lesions are seen in leishmaniasis. Persistent diarrhea and pneumonia can be the result of a number of infectious agents endemic in this region, although these symptoms are not seen in either acute or chronic Chagas disease.

206–210. The answers are: 206-A, 207-B, 208-C, 209-D, 210-E. *(Biochemistry of vitamins)* Phosphorylation of pyridoxine yields the biologically active form of vitamin B_6 (pyridoxal phosphate). This form serves as a coenzyme for a large number of enzymes, particularly those that catalyze reactions involving amino acids (e.g., transamination, deamination, decarboxylation, and condensation).

The biologically active form of folic acid is tetrahydrofolic acid. This form transfers one-carbon fragments to appropriate metabolites in the synthesis of amino acids, purines, and thymidylic acid, which is the characteristic pyrimidine of DNA.

Vitamin D_3 is converted to the active form, 1,25-dihydroxycholecalciferol, by two sequential hydroxylation reactions. The active form of vitamin D_3 stimulates the intestinal absorption of calcium and phosphate, increases the mobilization of calcium and phosphate from bone, and promotes the renal reabsorption of calcium and phosphate (in physiologic amounts).

The biologically active forms of niacin, or nicotinic acid, are nicotinamide adenine dinucleotide (NAD^+) and nicotinamide adenine dinucleotide phosphate ($NADP^+$). These two cofactors serve as coenzymes in oxidation–reduction reactions in which the coenzyme undergoes reduction of the pyridine ring by accepting a hydride ion (hydrogen ion plus one electron). The reduced forms of these two dinucleotides are NADH and NADPH, respectively.

Thiamine pyrophosphate is the biologically active form of vitamin B_1. It serves as a cofactor in the oxidative decarboxylation of keto acids. It is a cofactor in the nonoxidative reactions of the pentose phosphate pathway because it is the prosthetic group of transketolase.

211–214. The answers are: 211-C, 212-D, 213-A, 214-D. *(Diaphragm)* The aortic hiatus of the diaphragm transmits the aorta, the azygos vein, and the thoracic duct. The esophageal opening contains the esophagus and both vagus nerves. The vena caval foramen passes the inferior vena cava and the right phrenic nerve. The splanchnic nerves, the superior epigastric artery, and the hemiazygos vein pierce the crura separately.

215–218. The answers are: 215-E, 216-B, 217-C, 218-D. *(Respiratory histology)* The tracheal epithelium consists mainly of ciliated cells (A) and goblet cells (C). These ciliated cells move mucus and entrapped debris. The epithelium rests on a basement membrane (E). Beneath the basement membrane is a lamina propria with multicellular glands (B); beneath the lamina propria is cartilage (D).

219–222. The answers are: 219-A, 220-B, 221-B, 222-D. *(Anatomy of the small intestine)* Differences between segments of the small intestine are subtle; however, several distinguishing features aid identification. The jejunum contains well-developed plicae circulares, tall arteriae rectae, and few arterial arcades. The ileum has rudimentary plicae circulares, short arteriae rectae, and many arterial arcades. Meckel's diverticulum, a remnant of the embryonic vitelline duct, is present in the ileum in approximately 3% of the population. Appendices epiploicae (fat-filled tags) are diagnostic for the large bowel only.

223–226. The answers are: 223-B, 224-A, 225-C, 226-B. *(Embryology)* The fertilized egg, or zygote, gives rise to a morula, which in turn develops into a blastocyst. The embryoblast, or inner cell mass, is a loose collection of blastomeres bordering the blastocoele of the blastocyst. The trophoblast is an epithelial layer making up the wall of the blastocyst and surrounding the embryoblast. Thus, the zygote gives rise to both the embryoblast and the trophoblast. The trophoblast forms the cytotrophoblast and the syncytiotrophoblast; later in development, it forms the extraembryonic membranes such as the chorion and the bulk of the placenta as well. The epiblast and hypoblast are the two layers of the bilaminar disk–stage pre-embryo, and as such, like other structures comprising the body of the developing pre-embryo, are derived from the embryoblast.

227–230. The answers are: 227-B, 228-D, 229-C, 230-A. *(Skeletal disease)* Osteopetrosis, also known as Albers-Schönberg disease, is a hereditary disease characterized by the overgrowth and sclerosis of bone, resulting in thickening of the cortex and a narrowing of the medullary cavity. This disease is thought to be due to decreased osteoclast function. The juvenile form of osteopetrosis is usually lethal in utero or in the neonatal period. The adult form is relatively benign and results in anemia and a predisposition to bone factors.

Exostoses may occur as sporadic, solitary lesions or in great numbers in the autosomal dominant hereditary disorder osteochondromatosis. In this case, males are affected three times more often than females. Hereditary exostoses are not neoplasms but, rather, are developmentally misdirected projections of bone growth capped by cartilage. These growths of epiphyseal bone extend into the metaphyseal region and are found most often in the long bones of the extremities. Although benign, these lesions do have the potential for malignant transformation.

Achondroplasia is a form of dwarfism that results from premature ossification of epiphyseal plate cartilage. Heterozygous individuals with this form of dwarfism usually have normal intelligence, sexual development, and life span. Homozygosity for this genetic abnormality is usually fatal soon after birth.

Osteogenesis imperfecta, commonly called "brittle bone" disease, refers to a group of closely related disorders of type I collagen synthesis. As type I collagen comprises approximately 90% of bone matrix, these disorders result in marked thinning of bone cortex and reduced amounts of trabecular bone.

Osteoporosis is characterized by a reduction in bone mass, which may produce pain and increase vulnerability to fracture.

231–236. The answers are: 231-B, 232-B, 233-C, 234-C, 235-B, 236-A. *(Dermatology)* Eczema is a common name for a number of different conditions, including allergic contact dermatitis, atopic dermatitis, and primary irritant dermatitis. All are moist, red, papulovesicular lesions, which first become crusted and then develop elevated, scaling plaques. The edema fluid accumulates in and the vesicles arise from the intraepidermal–intraepithelial region.

Pemphigus vulgaris most often involves the mucosa and skin of the scalp, face, axilla, groin, and areas of skin subjected to pressure. The oral lesions often appear long before the skin lesions. The disease is an autoimmune disorder which causes the loss of attachment between epithelial cells; thus, this disease is also characterized by intraepithelial vesicles. A suprabasal acantholytic blister is present in pemphigus.

Pemphigoid is another fairly common autoimmune vesiculobullous disease. The vesicles, or rather blisters, are larger than those seen in pemphigus and are also less likely to rupture; thus pemphigoid blisters often heal without scarring. The immune abnormality consists of the linear deposition of immunoglobulin and complement in the basement membrane. Pemphigoid is a disease characterized by a subepidermal, nonacantholytic blister.

Patients with dermatitis herpetiformis often also present with celiac disease and express human leukocyte antigen (HLA) -B8 and HLA-DRw3 and develop IgA antibodies to dietary gluten (from wheat flour). These antibodies or immune complexes are then deposited in the skin and react with the anchoring fibrils of dermal papillae. Autoimmune damage to these dermal elements, in addition to the formation of microabscesses of neutrophils and eosinophils, results in the generation of subepithelial vesicles.

Darier's disease results from abnormal intraepithelial cross-bridging, including desmosomes. Due to these abnormalities, this disease manifests as regions of intraepithelial vesicles. Miliaria is a condition in which the sweat gland ducts are blocked, most usually by superficial epidermal infection. This results in the accumulation of fluid and subcorneal vesicle formation.

237–241. The answers are: 237-D, 238-A, 239-B, 240-E, 241-C. *(Female reproductive histology)* The diagram shows the organs in the female reproductive system. The vagina (A) has a stratified squamous unkeratinized epithelium. The vagina does not have glands; vaginal fluids are leakage from mucosal blood vessels. The cervix (B) has an epithelial transitional zone where the stratified squamous unkeratinized epithelium of the portion facing the vagina gives way to the simple columnar epithelium of the portion facing the uterus. The cervical canal has deep crypts that resemble glands. The uterus (C) and uterine tubes (E) are lined by simple columnar epithelium. Mucus-secreting cells predominate in the uterus, and ciliated cells predominate in the uterine tubes. The ovary (D) is coated with a simple cuboidal epithelium (germinal epithelium) that is continuous with the simple squamous epithelium (mesothelium) that lines the peritoneal cavity. The ovarian cortex consists of follicles containing gametogenic oocytes surrounded by stromal fibroblasts.

242–245. The answers are: 242-D, 243-C, 244-A, 245-B. *(Sensory receptors)* Merkel's cells are modified epidermal cells in the stratum basale. The terminal disk of an afferent nerve lies in close proximity to Merkel's cell to form a mechanoreceptor.

Meissner's corpuscles consist of an afferent nerve, flattened modified Schwann cells, spiral terminals of the afferent fiber, and a cellular collagenous capsule. They are responsible for fine touch and ususally are located in the dermal papillae of thick skin.

Pacini's corpuscles are ellipsoid, encapsulated sensory receptors that respond to pressure, vibration, and touch. A cross section of a pacinian corpuscle resembles an onion due to its concentrically laminated cells. They are primarily located in the dermis and hypodermis.

Ruffini's endings consist of a myelinated afferent nerve fiber that branches into multiple unmyelinated nerve terminals intertwined with collagen and encapsulated by a thin connective tissue. Ruffini's endings respond to pressure and touch and are found in skin and joints.

Krause's end bulbs consist of terminal branches of an afferent nerve fiber. They are spherical, surrounded by a thin cellular capsule, and primarily exist in mucous membranes.

246–250. The answers are: 246-E, 247-B, 248-B, 249-A, 250-A. *(Muscle innervation)* The spinal accessory nerve innervates the sternomastoid and trapezius muscles. The facial nerve innervates the muscles of facial expression, including the occipitofrontalis and platysma. The ansa cervicalis from C2 to C4 innervates the strap muscles, including the omohyoid and geniohyoid muscles. The greater auricular and lesser occipital nerves, as well as the greater occipital, transverse cervical, and supraclavicular nerves, are sensory branches of the cervical plexus.